EASY QUICK

HEALTHY

MEAL PREP COOKBOOK

Conquer Meal Prep: Quick, Freezer-Friendly, Make-Ahead Recipes for Busy People

DR JANE T. RYAN

INTRODUCTION

"Welcome to the culinary journey where convenience meets health in the pages of our Easy Quick Healthy Meal Prep Cookbook. Unleash the magic of effortless yet nutritious meals as we guide you through a collection of vibrant recipes designed to simplify your kitchen routine. Discover the art of efficient meal preparation without compromising on flavor or well-being. Let this cookbook be your companion in crafting delicious, time-saving, and wholesome dishes that make healthy eating a delightful and achievable lifestyle."

Overview of Meal Prep: Mastering Efficiency for Health and Flavor

In the realm of modern-day living, finding a harmonious balance between health and convenience can be a culinary challenge. Our Easy Quick Healthy Meal Prep Cookbook is your compass in navigating this journey. Let's delve into the heart of meal preparation, where efficiency becomes the cornerstone for fostering a healthier lifestyle.

1. The Essence of Meal Prep:

- Meal prep is not just about saving time – it's a strategic approach to fueling your body with nutrient-packed, delicious meals. We redefine the concept, emphasizing the art of planning, organizing, and preparing ahead to seamlessly integrate wholesome choices into your daily routine.

2. Health at the Core:

- Our cookbook is a celebration of health without compromise. Each recipe is meticulously crafted to ensure a perfect fusion of taste and nutrition. From vibrant salads to protein-rich mains, discover a spectrum of flavors that cater to your taste buds and well-being simultaneously.

3. Time-Saving Techniques:

- Unlock the secrets of efficient meal prep with our detailed guide on time-saving techniques. Learn to streamline your cooking process without sacrificing quality, empowering you to enjoy nourishing meals even on the busiest days.

4. Ingredient Mastery:

- Explore the variety of ingredients that form the foundation of our recipes. From fresh produce to lean proteins and wholesome grains, our cookbook embraces a diverse palette, proving that healthy eating is anything but monotonous.

5. Planning Made Easy:

- Embark on a journey of organized meal planning with our expert tips. Whether you're a seasoned meal prepper or just starting, our cookbook provides practical insights to simplify your weekly preparation, ensuring a stress-free and enjoyable cooking experience.

6. Culinary Creativity Unleashed:

- Meal prep is not a monotonous task but an opportunity to unleash your culinary creativity. Our cookbook encourages experimentation with flavors, textures, and cuisines, making each meal a delightful adventure in your own kitchen.
- In the pages that follow, let the Easy Quick Healthy Meal Prep Cookbook be your guide to a culinary world where health and flavor coexist effortlessly. Embrace the joy of preparing meals that not only nourish your body but also satisfy your taste buds, making the journey towards a healthier you an exciting and flavorsome expedition.

- Embarking on the journey of Easy Quick Healthy Meal Prep comes with a multitude of benefits, transforming the way you approach nutrition and well-being. As you dive into the pages of our cookbook, anticipate a myriad of advantages that extend beyond the kitchen.

1. Time Efficiency:

- Effortless meal prep translates into reclaimed time. By strategically planning and preparing your meals, you free up valuable hours in your week, allowing for a more balanced and stress-free lifestyle. Say goodbye to the rush and welcome the luxury of time.

2. Consistent Nutrient Intake:

- One of the key advantages of meal prep is the ability to maintain a consistent and balanced nutrient intake. Our cookbook guides you in crafting meals rich in essential vitamins, minerals, and macronutrients, ensuring your body receives the nourishment it deserves.

3. Weight Management Made Simple:

- Meal prep serves as a powerful tool in managing your weight. By controlling portion sizes and selecting wholesome ingredients, you empower yourself to make mindful choices, contributing to a sustainable and effective approach to weight management.

4. Financial Savings:

- Say farewell to impulsive food purchases and dining out expenses. Easy Quick Healthy Meal Prep is not just a culinary endeavor but a financial strategy. Experience the savings that come with buying ingredients in bulk, minimizing food waste, and curbing the temptation of pricey takeout options.

5. Enhanced Flavor Exploration:

- Our cookbook introduces you to a world of diverse and delectable flavors. Through strategic meal prep, you can experiment with a variety of herbs, spices, and ingredients, transforming each meal into a culinary adventure. Discover a newfound appreciation for the art of flavor without compromising on health.

6. Stress Reduction:

- Imagine a week where the question "What's for dinner?" is already answered. Easy Quick Healthy Meal Prep is a stress-reducing practice that eliminates the last-minute chaos of meal decisions. Experience a sense of calm knowing that nutritious and delicious options are readily available.

7. Customized Nutrition:

- Tailor your meals to meet your specific nutritional needs and dietary preferences. Our cookbook provides a diverse range of recipes, catering to various dietary lifestyles – from vegetarian and vegan to low-carb and high-protein. Personalize your plate with ease.

8. Long-term Health Benefits:

- Committing to Easy Quick Healthy Meal Prep isn't just about short-term gains; it's an investment in your long-term health. The consistency of nutritious eating contributes to improved energy levels, better immune function, and a reduced risk of chronic diseases.
- Incorporating the principles of Easy Quick Healthy Meal Prep into your culinary routine is not merely a choice – it's a transformative lifestyle decision. Embrace the multitude of benefits that extend far beyond the kitchen, paving the way for a healthier, more balanced, and enjoyable way of living.

CHAPTER I

GETTING STARTED

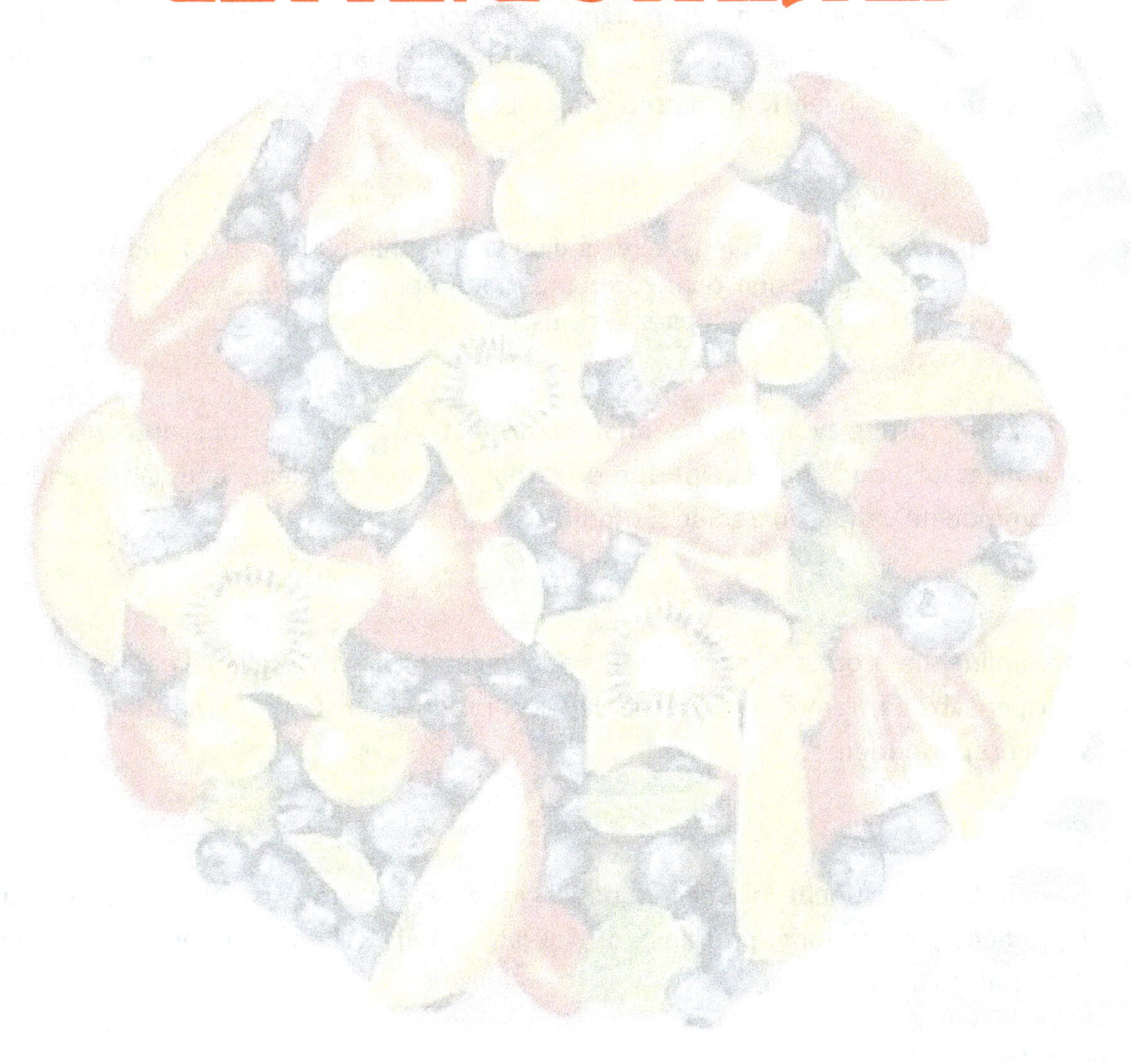

Essential Kitchen Tools for Easy, Quick, and Healthy Meal Prep

In the quest for efficient and health-conscious meal preparation, having the right kitchen tools is paramount. A well-equipped kitchen can significantly streamline the process of creating easy, quick, and nutritious meals. This guide outlines essential kitchen tools that are indispensable for anyone following a quick healthy meal prep cookbook.

Sharp Chef's Knife:

- Any well-prepared kitchen must have a chef's knife that is both sharp and of the highest caliber. It makes precision dicing, slicing, and chopping easier, which speeds up and improves the experience of preparing meals.

Cutting Board:

- A durable cutting board is essential to protect your countertops and maintain the sharpness of your knives. Opt for one that is easy to clean and large enough to accommodate various ingredients simultaneously.

Vegetable Peeler:

- Streamline the process of peeling fruits and vegetables with a reliable peeler. This tool is indispensable for removing the outer layer of produce, ensuring a smoother and quicker meal prep experience.

Mixing Bowls:

- Having an assortment of mixing bowls in different sizes is crucial for combining ingredients, marinating proteins, or tossing salads. Choose durable, easy-to-clean materials for convenience.

Non-Stick Pans:

- Non-stick pans are essential for cooking with minimal oil, promoting healthier meal options. Look for quality non-stick coatings to make clean-up a breeze.

Steamer Basket:

- For a quick and nutritious cooking method, invest in a steamer basket. It's perfect for preserving the nutrients in vegetables and proteins while achieving a tender texture.

- A powerful blender or food processor is a versatile tool for creating smoothies, sauces, and dressings. It's a time-saving solution for achieving the right consistency in your recipes.

Measuring Cups and Spoons:

- Precision is key in cooking, especially when following a recipe. Accurate measuring cups and spoons ensure that you achieve the perfect balance of ingredients for flavor and nutrition.

Instant-Read Thermometer:

- Cooking proteins to the right temperature is crucial for both safety and taste. An instant-read thermometer ensures your meals are cooked to perfection every time.

Baking Sheets:

- Ideal for roasting vegetables, baking proteins, or preparing healthy snacks, a reliable set of baking sheets is a must-have. Look for durable, non-stick options for easy cleaning.

Storage Containers:

- Simplify the process of portioning and storing your prepped meals by investing in high-quality, airtight storage containers. This promotes organization and allows for easy reheating.
- Equipping your kitchen with these essential tools lays the foundation for successful and efficient meal prep, especially when following an easy, quick, and healthy cookbook. From precise cutting to efficient cooking and convenient storage, these tools are your allies in creating delicious and nutritious meals with ease.

Smart Grocery Shopping Tips for Easy, Quick, and Healthy Meal Prep

Efficient and health-conscious meal preparation starts with smart grocery shopping. Planning and selecting the right ingredients are essential steps to ensure you can effortlessly follow an easy, quick, and healthy meal prep cookbook. This guide provides valuable tips to make your grocery shopping experience efficient and effective.

Plan Your Meals in Advance:

- Make a weekly meal plan before you shop for groceries. Review the recipes in your cookbook, create a shopping list, and stick to it. This minimizes impulse purchases and ensures you have everything you need.

Focus on Fresh Produce:

- Prioritize the fresh produce section. Opt for a variety of colorful fruits and vegetables, as they form the foundation of a healthy and balanced diet. Choose seasonal options for better flavor and cost-effectiveness.

Explore the Perimeter of the Store:

- Fresh produce, lean meats, and dairy are usually located around the perimeter of the grocery store. The majority of complete, unprocessed foods are found here. Reduce the amount of time you spend in the processed and packaged products aisles.

Choose Whole Grains:

- When selecting grains, opt for whole grains like quinoa, brown rice, and whole wheat pasta. These provide more nutrients and fiber, contributing to a healthier meal prep.

Include Lean Proteins:

- Incorporate lean proteins such as poultry, fish, tofu, and legumes into your shopping list. These protein sources are essential for muscle maintenance and overall well-being.

Read Labels Carefully:

- Read food labels carefully, especially if you are choosing packaged foods. Seek for items that are low in salt, have few ingredients, and have no added sugar. Maintaining a healthy diet requires knowing what is in your food.

Stock Up on Healthy Fats:

- Include sources of healthy fats in your shopping list, such as avocados, nuts, seeds, and olive oil. These fats are essential for overall health and can add flavor and richness to your meals.

Minimize Processed Foods:

- Don't overstock your cart with processed and prepackaged goods. Preservatives, bad fats, and added sugars are frequently found in these. Choose actual, whole foods to get the most nutritious value.

Consider Frozen and Canned Options:

- While fresh produce is ideal, frozen and canned fruits and vegetables can be convenient alternatives. They have a longer shelf life and are often just as nutritious. Choose options without added sugars or excessive salt.

Take Advantage of Sales and Discounts:

- Look out for specials, discounts, and bargains. You can save money by purchasing in bulk or by taking advantage of special offers, particularly on necessities.

Be Mindful of Portion Sizes:

- Be conscious of portion sizes, especially when purchasing snacks and treats. Avoid oversized packages, as they may lead to overeating.
- Smart grocery shopping lays the groundwork for successful and efficient meal prep when following an easy, quick, and healthy cookbook. By planning ahead, focusing on whole foods, and making informed choices, you'll not only save time but also support your journey towards a healthier lifestyle.

2week meal plan

Week 1:

Day 1:

- Breakfast: Avocado and Egg Breakfast Sandwich
- Lunch: Quinoa Salad with Roasted Vegetables
- Dinner: Chicken and Vegetable Stir-Fry

Day 2:

- Breakfast: Overnight Oats with Mixed Berries
- Lunch: Turkey and Avocado Wrap
- Dinner: Baked Salmon with Lemon and Dill

Day 3:

- Breakfast: Greek Yogurt Parfait with Granola
- Lunch: Vegetarian Chili with Black Beans
- Dinner: Sweet Potato and Chickpea Curry

Day 4:

- Breakfast: Energy Bites with Nuts and Dried Fruits
- Lunch: Hummus and Veggie Sticks
- Dinner: Sheet Pan Lemon Garlic Chicken with Vegetables

Day 5:

- Breakfast: Fruit Salad with Mint
- Lunch: Guacamole with Whole Grain Tortilla Chips
- Dinner: Shrimp and Broccoli Bake

Day 6:

- **Breakfast**: Greek Yogurt Popsicles
- **Lunch**: Veggie-Packed Frittata
- **Dinner**: Lentil and Spinach Stuffed Peppers

Day 7:

- **Breakfast**: Dark Chocolate-Dipped Strawberries
- **Lunch**: Mushroom and Spinach Quiche
- **Dinner**: Spinach and Feta Chickpea Patties

Day 8:

- **Breakfast**: Zucchini Noodles with Pesto
- **Lunch**: Cauliflower Fried Rice
- **Dinner**: Turkey and Vegetable Lettuce Wraps

Day 9:

- **Breakfast**: Teriyaki Chicken Bowls
- **Lunch**: Quick and Easy Shrimp Scampi
- **Dinner**: Beef and Broccoli Stir-Fry

Day 10:

- **Breakfast**: Chicken and Rice Casserole
- **Lunch**: Vegetarian Lasagna Roll-Ups
- **Dinner**: Black Bean and Corn Quesadillas

You can mix and match these to suit your dietary requirements and tastes!

CHAPTER 2

BREAKFAST RECIPES

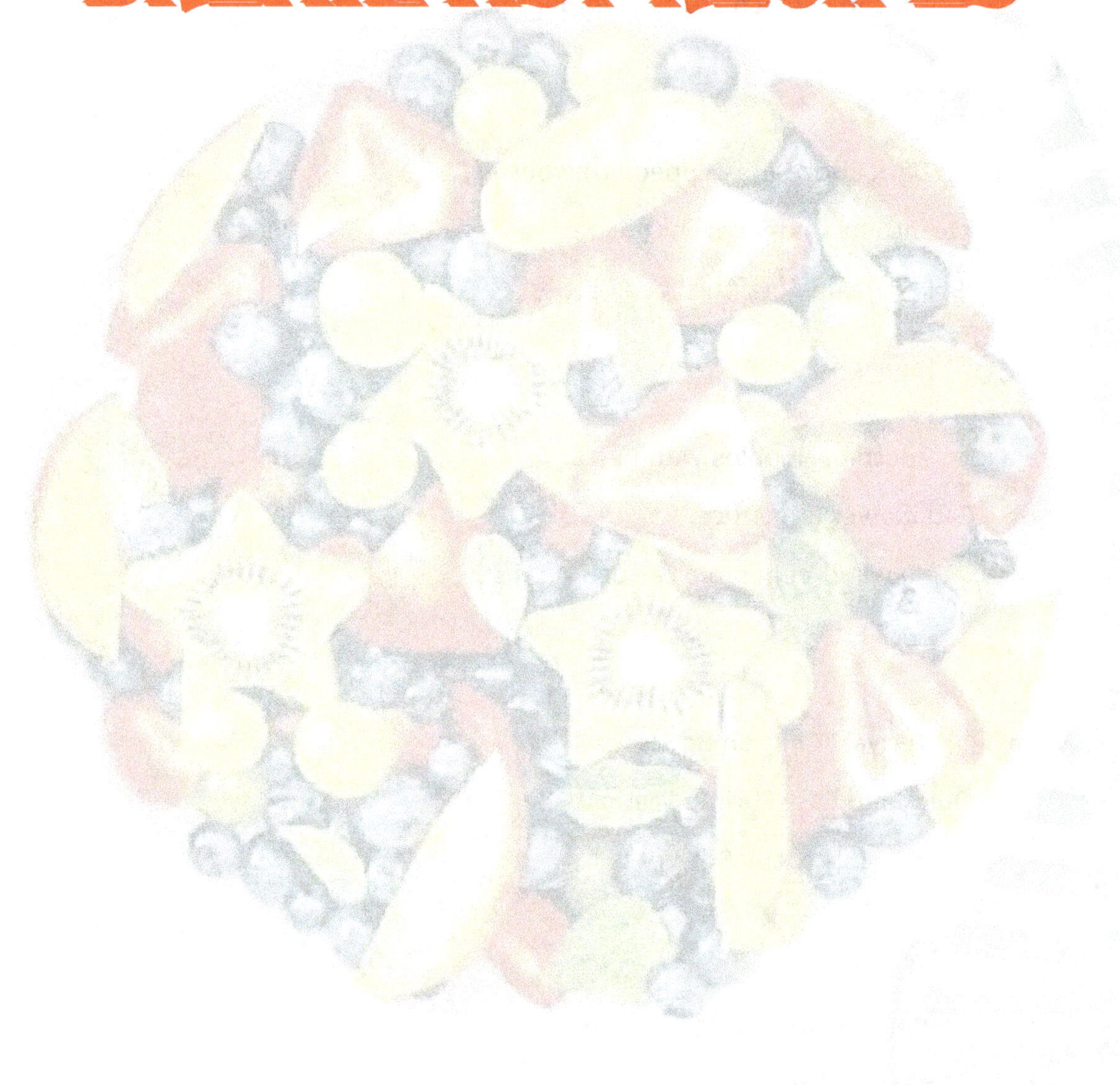

Avocado and Egg Breakfast Sandwich

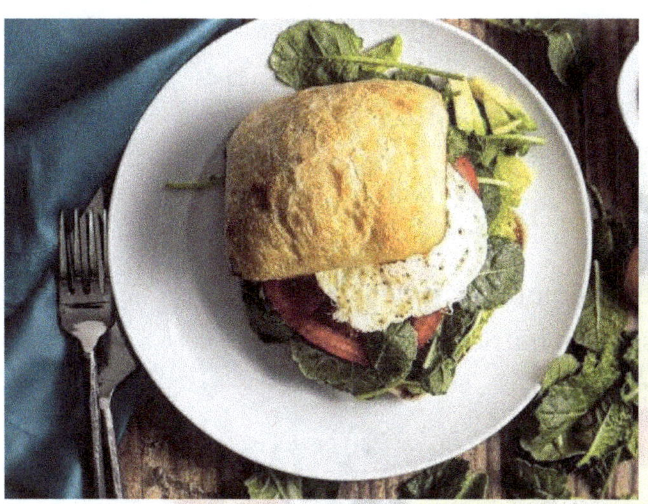

Ingredients:

- 2 slices of whole-grain bread
- 1 ripe avocado
- 2 large eggs
- Salt and pepper to taste
- Optional toppings: sliced tomatoes, red onion, or cheese

Procedure:

- As desired, toast the slices of whole-grain bread.
- Mash the ripe avocado in a bowl and season with salt and pepper while toasted.
- In a non-stick pan, cook the eggs as per your preference (fried, scrambled, or poached).
- Spread the mashed avocado evenly on one side of each toasted bread slice.
- Place the cooked eggs on one bread slice and add optional toppings if desired.
- Place the second slice of bread on top to form a sandwich.

Time of Preparation:

- Approximately 15 minutes.

Tips and Tricks:

- Choose ripe avocados for a creamy texture.
- Experiment with different egg preparations for variety.

- For an added heat, add a splash of salsa or hot sauce.

- Calories: Approximately 400-500
- Protein: 15-20g
- Healthy fats: 20-25g
- Fiber: 8-10g

Health Benefits:

- Avocados: high in heart-healthy fats, they promote heart health.
- Eggs provide high-quality protein and essential nutrients.
- Whole-grain bread adds fiber, aiding digestion.

Packaging and Storing:

- Best enjoyed fresh; however, you can prepare components ahead and assemble just before eating.
- Store any leftover avocado mix in an airtight container to prevent browning.

Estimated Cost of Preparation:

- Depending on the quality of ingredients, approximately $5-$8 per serving.

Precautions:

- Be cautious while handling the knife and hot cooking surfaces.
- Check for egg allergies before serving to individuals with dietary restrictions.

Post-Caution:

- Refrigerate any leftover sandwich components promptly.
- Reheat eggs cautiously to avoid overcooking.

Overnight Oats with Mixed Berries

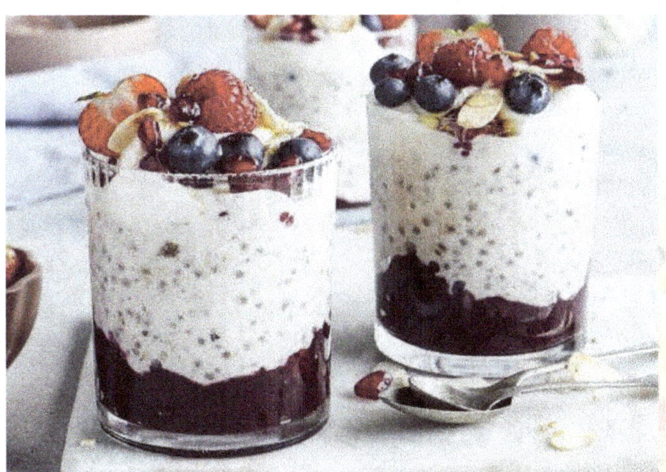

Ingredients:

- 1/2 cup rolled oats
- 1/2 cup milk (dairy or plant-based)
- 1/2 cup mixed berries (strawberries, blueberries, raspberries)
- 1 tablespoon chia seeds
- 1 tablespoon honey or maple syrup
- 1/2 teaspoon vanilla extract
- Optional toppings: nuts, yogurt, or additional berries

Procedure:

- In a jar or container, combine rolled oats, milk, mixed berries, chia seeds, honey or maple syrup, and vanilla extract.
- For all ingredients to be dispersed equally, give it a good stir. Refrigerate the jar or container for at least 6 to 8 hours after sealing it. Give the mixture a brisk toss in the morning and adjust with desired toppings.

Time of Preparation:

- 5 minutes (plus overnight refrigeration).

Tips and Tricks:

- Use a jar with a lid for easy storage and portability.
- Experiment with different milk alternatives for varied flavors.

- Adjust sweetness to taste; you can add more honey or maple syrup if desired.

Nutritional Value per Serving:

- Calories: Approximately 300-350
- Protein: 8-10g
- Fiber: 10-12g
- Antioxidants from mixed berries

Health Benefits:

- Oats provide a good source of fiber and sustained energy.
- Berries are rich in antioxidants and vitamins.
- Chia seeds provide extra fibre and omega-3 fatty acids..

Packaging and Storing:

- Prepare multiple jars for a week's worth of breakfasts.
- Keep refrigerated and consume within 3-4 days for optimal freshness.

Estimated Cost of Preparation:

- Around $3-$5 per serving, depending on the cost of berries and other ingredients.

Precautions:

- Check for allergies to any specific berries or seeds.
- Ensure the container is sealed properly to prevent spills in the refrigerator.

Post-Caution:

- If the texture is too thick in the morning, add a splash of milk and stir.
- Discard any jars that show signs of spoilage or an off smell.

Greek Yogurt Parfait with Granola

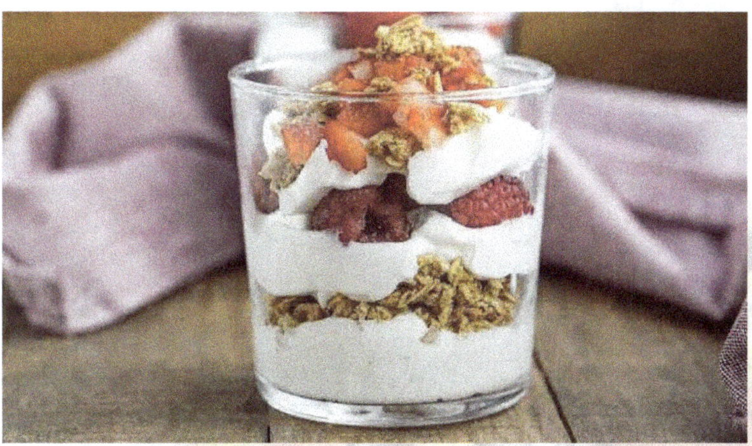

Ingredients:

- 1 cup Greek yogurt
- 1/2 cup granola (store-bought or homemade)
- 1/2 cup mixed fresh berries (strawberries, blueberries, or raspberries)
- 1 tablespoon honey or maple syrup
- 1/4 cup chopped nuts (e.g., almonds or walnuts)
- Optional: a sprinkle of cinnamon or a drizzle of nut butter

Procedure:

- In a glass or bowl, start with a layer of Greek yogurt.
- Add a layer of granola, followed by a layer of mixed berries.
- Layers should be repeated until the container is full.
- Drizzle honey or maple syrup over the top and sprinkle with chopped nuts.
- Optionally, add a dash of cinnamon or a drizzle of nut butter for extra flavor.

Time of Preparation:

- Approximately 5-10 minutes.

Tips and Tricks:

- Choose plain Greek yogurt for a healthier option and control sweetness with honey or maple syrup.
- Experiment with different granola flavors to suit your taste.

- Customize with additional toppings like coconut flakes or dark chocolate.

- Calories: Approximately 350-400
- Protein: 20-25g
- Healthy fats: 15-20g
- Fiber: 5-8g

Health Benefits:

- Probiotics and protein abound in Greek yoghurt.
- Berries offer antioxidants and vitamins.
- Nuts provide healthy fats and additional protein.

Packaging and Storing:

- Best enjoyed fresh; however, you can prepare components ahead and assemble just before eating.
- Keep refrigerated if preparing in advance.

Estimated Cost of Preparation:

- Around $4-$6 per serving, depending on the cost of Greek yogurt and berries.

Precautions:

- Be cautious if you have nut allergies; consider omitting nuts or choosing allergy-friendly alternatives.
- Check the granola ingredients for added sugars.

Post-Caution:

- Consume promptly after assembly to maintain granola crunchiness.
- Store any leftover components separately to prevent sogginess.

CHAPTER 3

LUNCH RECIPES

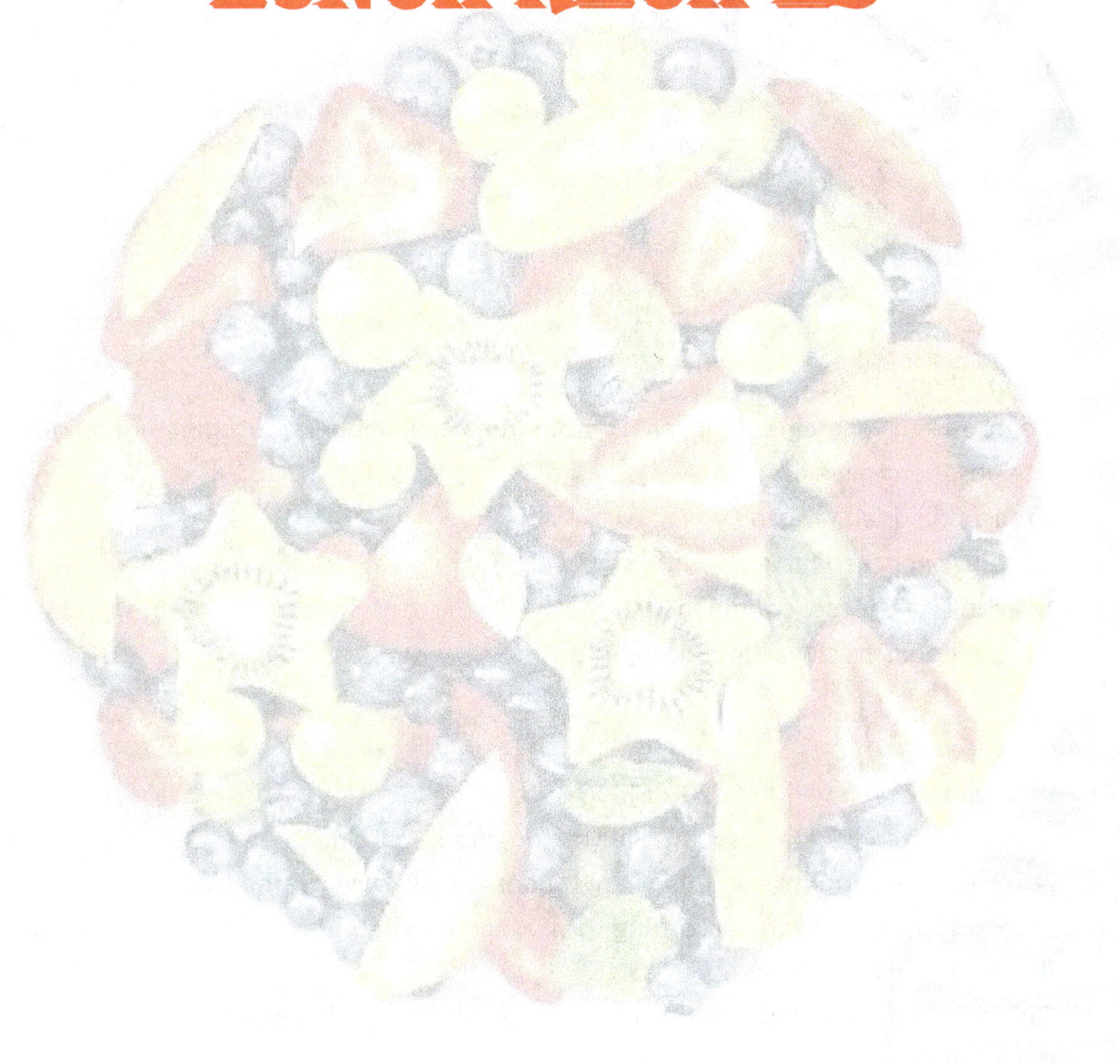

Quinoa Salad with Roasted Vegetables

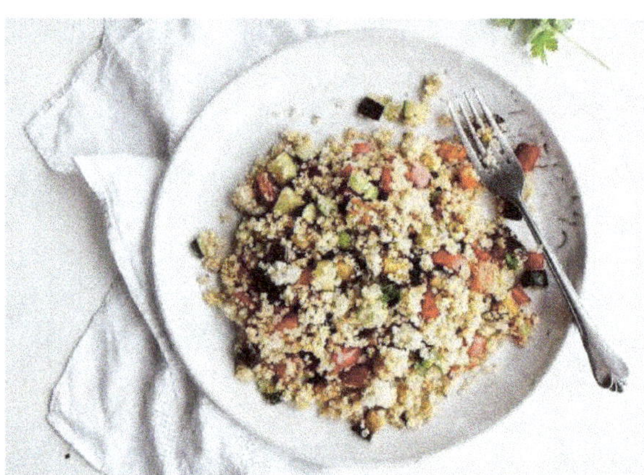

Ingredients:

- 1 cup quinoa, rinsed
- 2 cups mixed vegetables (e.g., cherry tomatoes, bell peppers, zucchini, red onion)
- 3 tablespoons olive oil
- 1 teaspoon dried oregano
- Salt and pepper to taste
- 1/4 cup feta cheese, crumbled
- 2 tablespoons fresh parsley, chopped

Procedures:

- Preheat the oven to 400°F (200°C).
- Toss the mixed vegetables with olive oil, oregano, salt, and pepper. Roast in the oven for 20-25 minutes or until vegetables are tender and slightly caramelized.
- Meanwhile, cook quinoa according to package instructions. After cooking, use a fork to fluff it up and let it to cool.
- Quinoa and the roasted veggies should be combined in a big bowl.
- Mix well.
- Add crumbled feta and chopped parsley. Toss gently to combine.
- Adjust seasoning if necessary. Serve chilled or at room temperature.

Time of Preparation:

- Approximately 40 minutes

- Rinse quinoa thoroughly to remove any bitterness.
- Tailor the veggie mixture to your individual tastes.
- Drizzle with balsamic glaze for extra flavor.

Nutritional Value per Serving:

- Calories: ~350
- Protein: ~10g
- Fiber: ~8g
- Healthy fats from olive oil.

Health Benefits:

- Rich in protein, fiber, and essential nutrients.
- Provides a good balance of carbohydrates for sustained energy.
- Supports heart health and weight management.

Packaging and Storing:

- For up to three days, keep in the refrigerator in an airtight container.
- Ideal for meal prepping; divide into portions for quick, healthy lunches.

Estimated Cost of Preparation:

- Approximately $15, depending on ingredient quality and location.

Precautions:

- Be cautious with salt; feta cheese adds saltiness.
- Ensure quinoa is cooked thoroughly for optimal texture.

Post-Caution:

- Monitor portion sizes for those watching caloric intake.
- Consider allergens if serving to guests.

Chicken and Vegetable Stir-Fry

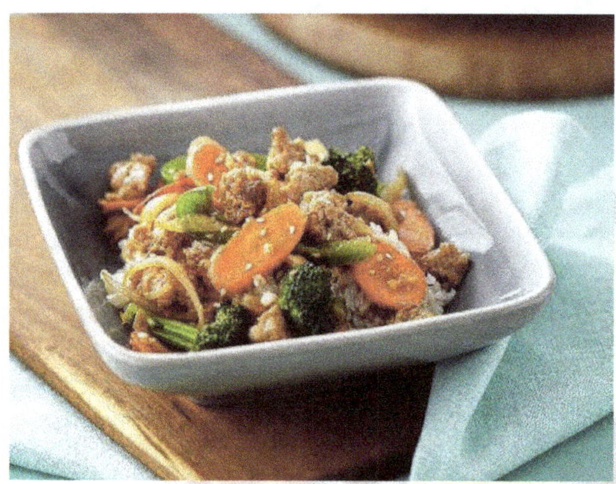

Ingredients:

- One pound (450g) of skinless, boneless chicken breasts, thinly sliced; three cups of mixed veggies, such as carrots, bell peppers, broccoli, and snap peas
- 2 tablespoons soy sauce
- 1 tablespoon oyster sauce
- 1 tablespoon hoisin sauce
- 2 tablespoons vegetable oil
- 2 cloves garlic, minced
- 1 teaspoon ginger, grated
- 2 green onions, sliced
- 1 tablespoon sesame seeds (optional)
- Cooked rice or noodles for serving

Procedures:

- In a wok or sizable skillet, heat the vegetable oil over medium-high heat.
- Add sliced chicken and stir-fry until browned and cooked through. Take out of the wok and place aside.
- If necessary, add a little extra oil to the same wok.
- Stir-fry garlic and ginger until fragrant.
- Add mixed vegetables and stir-fry until they are tender-crisp.
- Return the cooked chicken to the wok. Pour in soy sauce, oyster sauce, and hoisin sauce. Toss everything together until well-coated.

- Stir in sliced green onions and sesame seeds if desired.
- Serve the stir-fry with noodles or cooked rice.

Time of Preparation:

- Approximately 25 minutes

Tips and Tricks:

- Slice chicken thinly for faster cooking.
- Use a variety of colorful vegetables for a visually appealing dish.
- Add a splash of water if the wok gets too dry.

Nutritional Value per Serving:

- Calories: ~400
- Protein: ~30g
- Healthy fats from sesame seeds and vegetable oil.

Health Benefits:

- High in protein, essential vitamins, and minerals.
- gives a healthy ratio of fats and carbohydrates.
- Supports muscle development and overall well-being.

Packaging and Storing:

- Remaining food can be kept in the refrigerator for up to two days if it is sealed tightly.
- Reheat in a skillet or microwave for a quick and convenient meal.

Estimated Cost of Preparation:

- Approximately $20, depending on ingredient quality and location.

Precautions:

- Be cautious with soy sauce; it can be salty.
- Adjust sauce quantities based on personal taste preferences.

Post-Caution:

- Be mindful of portion sizes, especially if watching sodium intake.
- Experiment with different vegetables for variety.

Turkey and Avocado Wrap

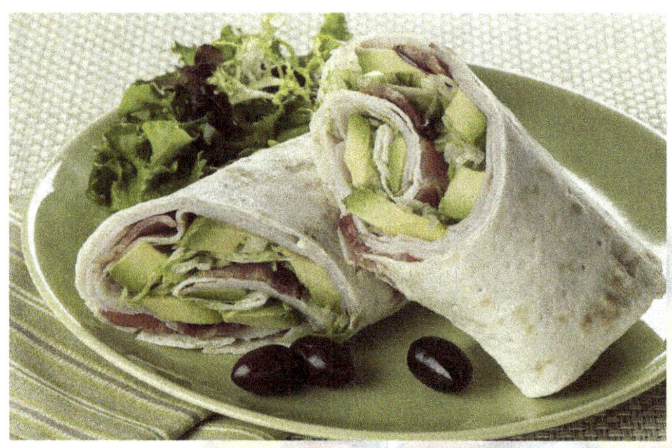

Ingredients:

- 8 oz (225g) sliced turkey breast
- 1 ripe avocado, sliced
- 1 cup cherry tomatoes, halved
- 1 cup lettuce, shredded
- 4 whole wheat or spinach wraps
- 1/4 cup plain Greek yogurt
- 2 tablespoons Dijon mustard
- Salt and pepper to taste

Procedures:

- Lay out the wraps and spread a thin layer of Greek yogurt on each one.
- In the center of each wrap, layer sliced turkey, avocado, cherry tomatoes, and shredded lettuce.
- Drizzle Dijon mustard over the fillings and season with salt and pepper to taste.
- Fold in the sides of the wrap and then roll tightly from the bottom to form a wrap.
- Slice in half diagonally and secure with toothpicks if needed.
- Serve right away or pack in parchment paper for a supper you can take with you.

Time of Preparation:

- Approximately 15 minutes

Tips and Tricks:

- Choose ripe avocados for creaminess.

- Warm the wraps briefly for added flexibility.
- Customize with your favorite veggies or add a sprinkle of cheese.

Nutritional Value per Serving:

- Calories: ~400
- Protein: ~25g
- Healthy fats from avocado and turkey.
- High in fiber from whole wheat wraps.

Health Benefits:

- wholesome supply of lean protein for muscles
- Avocado provides heart-healthy monounsaturated fats.
- Whole wheat wraps offer complex carbohydrates for sustained energy.

Packaging and Storing:

- Refrigerated for up to 24 hours, but best enjoyed fresh.
- To prevent sogginess, pack wet ingredients separately and assemble before eating.

Estimated Cost of Preparation:

- Approximately $15, depending on ingredient quality and location.

Precautions:

- Be cautious with condiment quantities; adjust to personal taste.
- Check turkey slices for added sodium; choose low-sodium options if necessary.

Post-Caution:

- Consider adding a squeeze of lemon to avocado slices to prevent browning.
- Monitor portions for those watching caloric or sodium intake.

CHAPTER 4

DINNER RECIPES

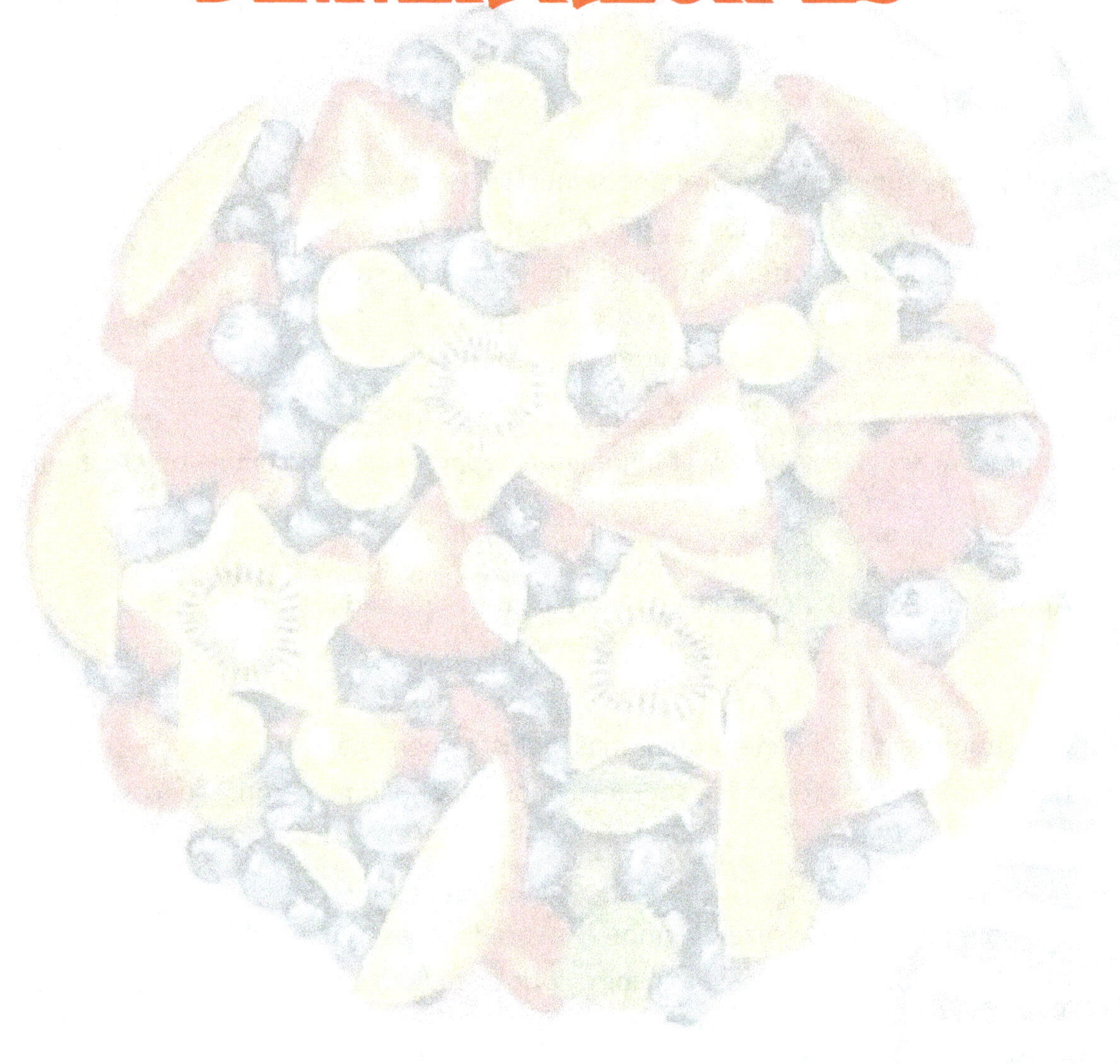

Baked Salmon with Lemon and Dill

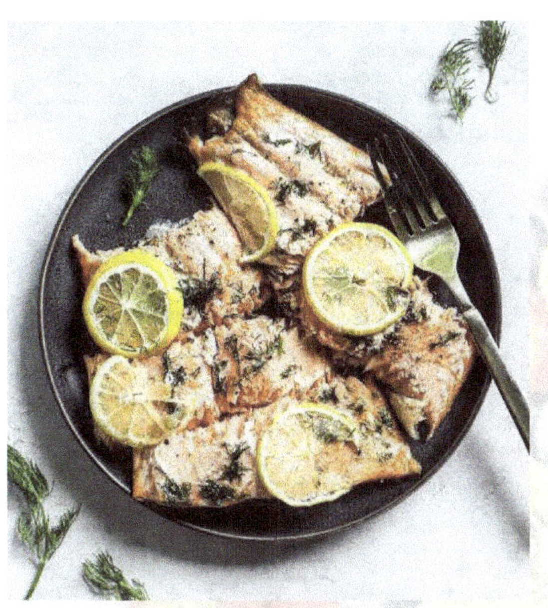

Ingredients:

- 4 salmon fillets
- 2 lemons (1 sliced, 1 juiced)
- 2 tablespoons olive oil
- 2 cloves garlic, minced
- 2 tablespoons fresh dill, chopped
- Salt and pepper to taste

Procedure:

- Preheat the oven to 400°F (200°C).
- Put the salmon fillets on a parchment paper-lined baking sheet.In a small bowl, mix together olive oil, minced garlic, lemon juice, chopped dill, salt, and pepper.
- Make sure the salmon fillets are evenly coated by brushing them with the lemon-dill mixture.
- Arrange lemon slices on top of each fillet for added flavor.
- Bake for 15 to 20 minutes, or until the salmon is cooked through and flake readily with a fork, in an oven that has been warmed.

- Approximately 30 minutes.

- Pat the salmon fillets dry before applying the marinade for better absorption.
- Adjust baking time based on the thickness of the fillets to prevent overcooking.

- Salmon is high in protein, vitamin D, and omega-3 fatty acids.
- Lemons provide vitamin C and antioxidants.
- Dill adds vitamins A and C.

- Supports heart health due to omega-3 fatty acids.
- Boosts immune system with vitamin C.
- Provides anti-inflammatory properties.

- Remaining food can be kept in the refrigerator for up to two days if it is sealed tightly.
- For longer storage, freeze the cooked salmon in a freezer-safe bag for up to 2 months.

- Cost varies based on salmon quality and local prices, but it's generally moderate.

- Ensure salmon is cooked thoroughly to avoid foodborne illness.
- Be cautious when handling hot pans and use oven mitts.

- Check for bones while eating.
- Consider sustainability when purchasing salmon.

Vegetarian Chili with Black Beans

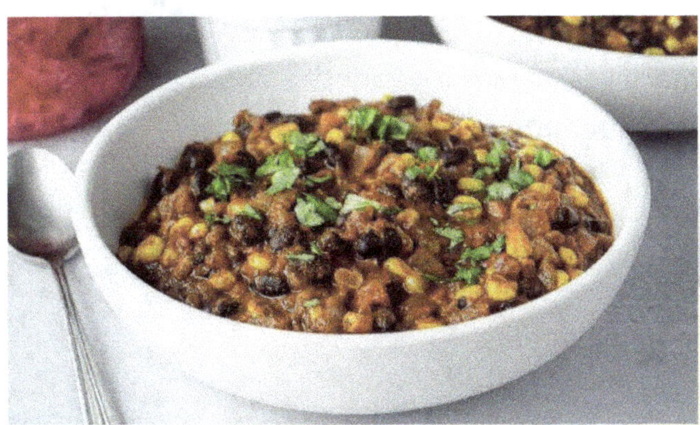

Ingredients:

- Two cans (15 oz each) of rinsed and drained black beans
- 1 can (28 oz) crushed tomatoes
- 1 large onion, chopped
- 1 bell pepper, diced
- 2 carrots, peeled and diced
- 3 cloves garlic, minced
- 1 cup corn kernels (fresh or frozen)
- 1 tablespoon olive oil
- 2 tablespoons chili powder
- 1 teaspoon cumin
- 1 teaspoon paprika
- Salt and pepper to taste
- Topping options include chopped green onions, sour cream, and shredded cheese.

Procedure:

- Heat the olive oil in a big pot over medium heat. Add the bell pepper, onions, and carrots. Sauté the veggies till they get soft.
- Add the paprika, cumin, chilli powder, minced garlic, salt, and pepper. Once fragrant, stir and simmer for one to two minutes.
- Pour in crushed tomatoes, black beans, and corn. Stir well.
- Bring the chili to a simmer, then reduce heat and let it cook uncovered for 20-25 minutes, stirring occasionally.
- To get the right consistency, add extra water if necessary and adjust the flavour to taste.

- Approximately 45 minutes.

Tips and Tricks:

- Experiment with different beans or add more vegetables for variety.
- Allow the chili to sit for a while before serving to enhance flavors.

Nutritional Value per Serving:

- High in fiber from black beans and vegetables.
- Packed with vitamins and antioxidants from vegetables.

Health Benefits:

- Plant-based protein from black beans.
- Low in fat and cholesterol.
- Supports digestion with fiber-rich ingredients.

Packaging and Storing:

- For up to four days, store in the refrigerator in sealed containers.
- Freeze in portions for longer storage, up to 3 months.

Estimated Cost of Preparation:

- Budget-friendly, as it primarily consists of pantry staples and vegetables.

Precautions:

- Be cautious with chili powder quantity; adjust to taste preference and spice tolerance.

Post-Caution:

- Consider adding dairy-free toppings for a vegan option.
- Monitor sodium levels, especially if using canned beans.

Sweet Potato and Chickpea Curry

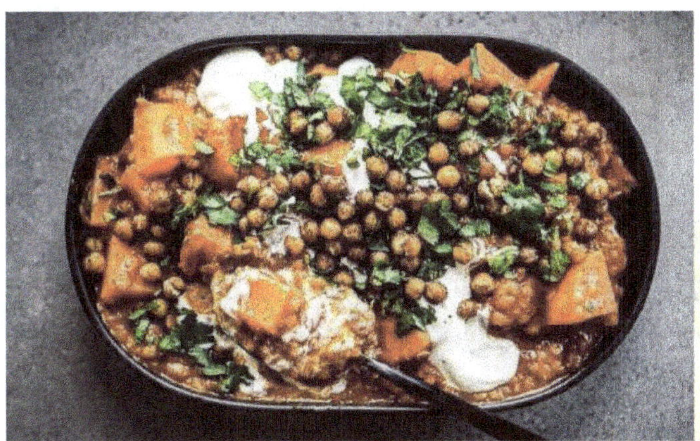

Ingredients:

- 2 medium sweet potatoes, peeled and cubed
- One can (15 oz) of rinsed and drained chickpeas
- 1 onion, finely chopped
- 3 cloves garlic, minced
- 1 can (14 oz) coconut milk
- 1 can (14 oz) diced tomatoes
- 1 cup vegetable broth
- 2 tablespoons curry powder
- 1 teaspoon ground turmeric
- 1 teaspoon ground cumin
- 1 teaspoon paprika
- 1 tablespoon olive oil
- Salt and pepper to taste
- Fresh cilantro for garnish

Procedure:

- Warm up the olive oil in a big pot over medium heat. Cook the chopped onions until they become tender.
- Add minced garlic, curry powder, ground turmeric, ground cumin, and paprika. Stir for 1-2 minutes until fragrant.
- Add sweet potatoes, chickpeas, diced tomatoes, coconut milk, and vegetable broth. Season with salt and pepper.

- After bringing the mixture to a boil, lower the heat so that it simmers. . Cover and cook for 20-25 minutes or until sweet potatoes are tender.
- Adjust seasoning if necessary and garnish with fresh cilantro before serving.

- Approximately 45 minutes.

- To change the amount of spiciness, add more or less curry powder.
- For a creamier texture, mash some sweet potatoes into the curry.

- High in fiber and plant-based protein from chickpeas.
- Rich in vitamins A and C from sweet potatoes.

- Supports digestive health with fiber from chickpeas and sweet potatoes.
- Anti-inflammatory properties from turmeric.
- Provides energy with complex carbohydrates from sweet potatoes.

- Store in airtight containers in the refrigerator for up to 3-4 days.
- This curry freezes well; divide into portions and freeze for up to 3 months.

- Affordable, as it mainly consists of budget-friendly ingredients.

- Be mindful of spice levels; adjust to personal preference.
- Ensure sweet potatoes are cooked through to achieve the desired tenderness.

- Consider serving with brown rice or whole-grain naan for a complete meal.
- Monitor portion sizes due to the richness of coconut milk.

CHAPTER 5

SNACK RECIPES

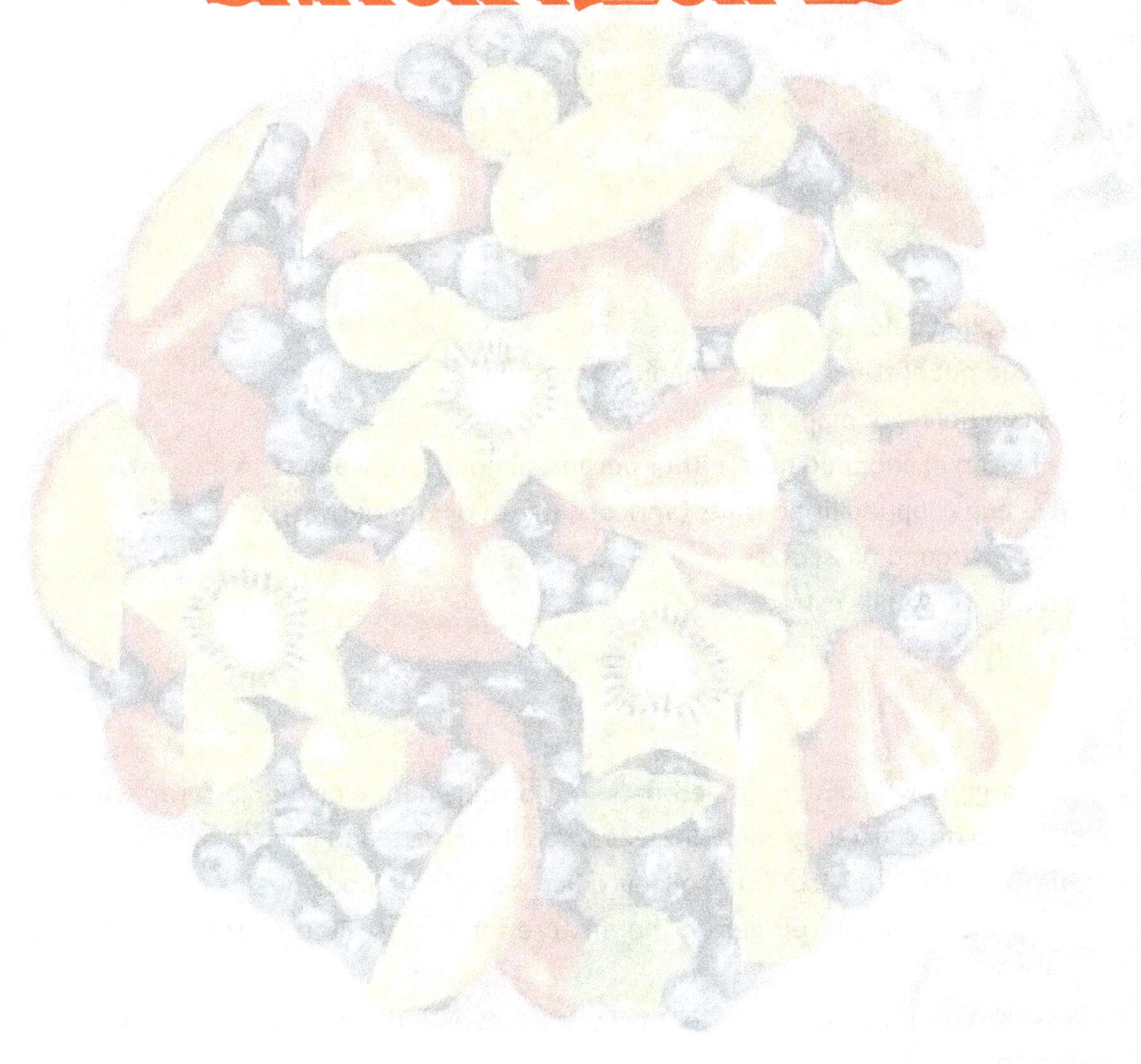

Energy Bites with Nuts and Dried Fruits

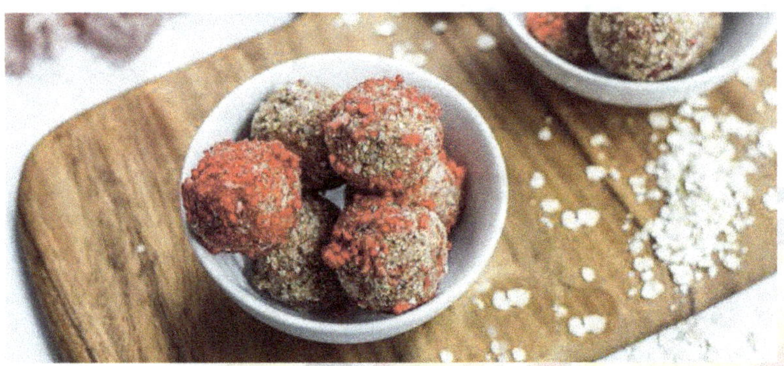

Ingredients:

- 1 cup rolled oats
- 1/2 cup nut butter (almond, peanut, or cashew)
- 1/3 cup honey or maple syrup
- Half a cup of chopped nuts, either pecans, almonds, or walnuts
- G1/2 cup chopped dried fruits (apricots, dates, or cranberries)
- 1/4 cup ground flaxseeds
- 1 teaspoon vanilla extract
- A pinch of salt

Procedure:

- In a large bowl, combine rolled oats, nut butter, honey or maple syrup, chopped nuts, chopped dried fruits, ground flaxseeds, vanilla extract, and a pinch of salt.
- Stir thoroughly to ensure that all ingredients are combined equally.
- Cover the bowl and refrigerate the mixture for at least 30 minutes to make it easier to handle.
- After the mixture has cold, take small quantities and use your hands to roll them into bite-sized balls.
- Place the energy bites on a parchment paper-lined tray and refrigerate for an additional 15-20 minutes to firm up.
- Store the energy bites in an airtight container in the refrigerator for freshness.

Time of Preparation:

- Approximately 15-20 minutes of active preparation time, plus chilling time.

- Customize the recipe by adding chia seeds, coconut flakes, or dark chocolate chips.
- Adjust sweetness by varying the amount of honey or maple syrup according to taste.

Nutritional Value per Serving:

- Calories: ~120-150 kcal per energy bite
- Rich in fiber, healthy fats, protein, and various vitamins and minerals.

Health Benefits:

- Provides a quick energy boost, ideal for pre- or post-workout snacks.
- Nutrient-dense ingredients support overall health, including heart health and digestion.

Packaging and Storing:

- For up to two weeks, keep in the refrigerator in an airtight container.
- Can be frozen for longer storage; thaw before consuming.

Estimated Cost of Preparation:

- Costs may vary based on the quality of ingredients and location. Generally budget-friendly.

Precautions:

- Check for allergies before serving, especially if nuts or other ingredients pose a risk.
- Be mindful with serving sizes to prevent consuming too many calories.

Post-Caution:

- Savour sparingly as part of a well-balanced diet.
- Experiment with ingredient ratios to find the perfect flavor and texture for your taste.

Hummus and Veggie Sticks

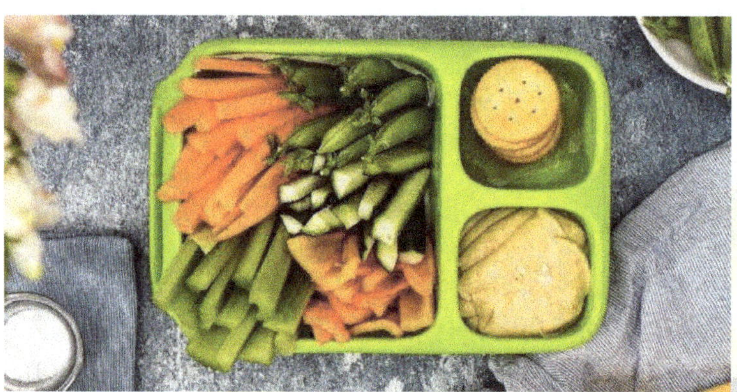

Ingredients:

- One can (15 oz) of rinsed and drained chickpeas
- 1/4 cup tahini
- 3 tablespoons olive oil
- 3 tablespoons lemon juice
- 2 cloves garlic, minced
- 1/2 teaspoon cumin
- Salt and pepper to taste
- Water (as needed for consistency)
- Assorted veggies for dipping (carrots, cucumbers, bell peppers, etc.)

Procedure:

- In a food processor, combine chickpeas, tahini, olive oil, lemon juice, minced garlic, cumin, salt, and pepper.
- Blend until smooth, adding water gradually to achieve the desired consistency.
- Taste and adjust seasoning as needed.
- Transfer the hummus to a serving bowl.
- Wash, peel, and cut assorted veggies into sticks for dipping.
- Serve the hummus with the veggie sticks.

Time of Preparation:

- Approximately 15-20 minutes.

- Add a pinch of smoked paprika or a drizzle of extra virgin olive oil for extra flavor.
- Adjust lemon juice and garlic to suit your taste preferences.

Nutritional Value per Serving:

- Hummus: ~70-80 kcal per 2 tablespoons
- Rich in protein, fiber, healthy fats, and various vitamins and minerals.

Health Benefits:

- Supports heart health due to healthy fats and fiber.
- Provides plant-based protein and nutrients.

Packaging and Storing:

- For up to a week, keep hummus refrigerated in an airtight container.
- Stir before serving if separation occurs.

Estimated Cost of Preparation:

- Cost-effective, with most ingredients being pantry staples.

Precautions:

- Be cautious of allergies, especially if guests have sesame or garlic allergies.
- Store veggie sticks properly to maintain freshness.

Post-Caution:

- Hummus can be a healthy addition to a balanced diet.
- Vary the veggie selection for a colorful and nutrient-rich snack.

Guacamole with Whole Grain Tortilla Chips

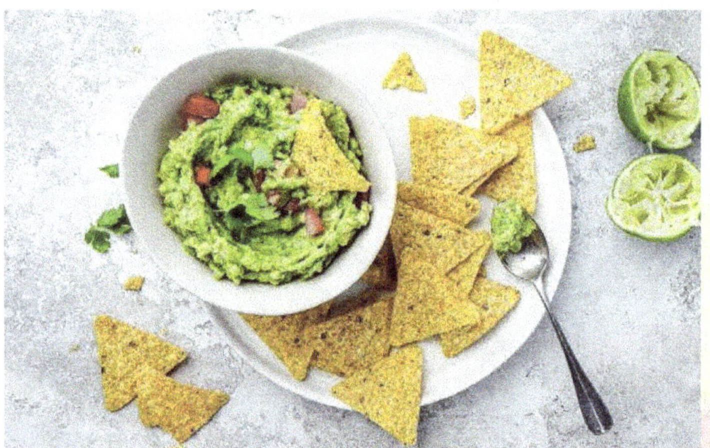

- For Guacamole:
- 3 ripe avocados
- 1 medium-sized tomato, diced
- 1/4 cup red onion, finely chopped
- 1/4 cup cilantro, chopped
- 1-2 cloves garlic, minced
- 1 lime, juiced
- Salt and pepper to taste
- For Whole Grain Tortilla Chips:
- Whole grain tortillas
- Olive oil spray
- Salt to taste

Procedure:

For Guacamole:

- Remove the pits from the avocados, cut them in half, and scoop out the meat into a bowl.
- Mash the avocados with a fork until smooth or leave it slightly chunky, depending on your preference.
- Add diced tomatoes, chopped red onion, cilantro, minced garlic, lime juice, salt, and pepper. Mix well.
- Taste and adjust the seasoning as needed.

- To keep the guacamole from browning, cover it with plastic wrap, making sure it contacts the surface.
- For Whole Grain Tortilla Chips:
- Preheat the oven to 350°F (175°C).
- Brush whole grain tortillas with olive oil or spray with olive oil spray.
- Sprinkle with salt and cut into triangles.
- Place on a baking sheet and bake for 10-12 minutes or until crisp.

Time of Preparation:

- Approximately 20-30 minutes.

Tips and Tricks:

- A dash of cayenne pepper can be added for extra heat.
- Keep the avocado pit in the guacamole to help prevent browning.

Nutritional Value per Serving:

- Guacamole: ~150-200 kcal per 1/2 cup serving
- Whole Grain Tortilla Chips: ~80-100 kcal per 1 oz serving

Health Benefits:

- Avocados provide healthy monounsaturated fats and essential nutrients.
- Whole grain tortillas offer fiber, promoting digestive health.

Packaging and Storing:

- Guacamole is best enjoyed fresh but can be stored in an airtight container in the refrigerator for up to a day.
- Store whole grain tortilla chips in a sealed bag or container to maintain crispness.

Estimated Cost of Preparation:

- Affordable, with basic and readily available ingredients.

Precautions:

- Be cautious with the amount of salt; avocados and tortilla chips may already have salt.
- Serve guacamole promptly to avoid discoloration.

- Guacamole is a nutritious dip suitable for various occasions.
- Experiment with different whole grain tortilla brands for varying flavors.

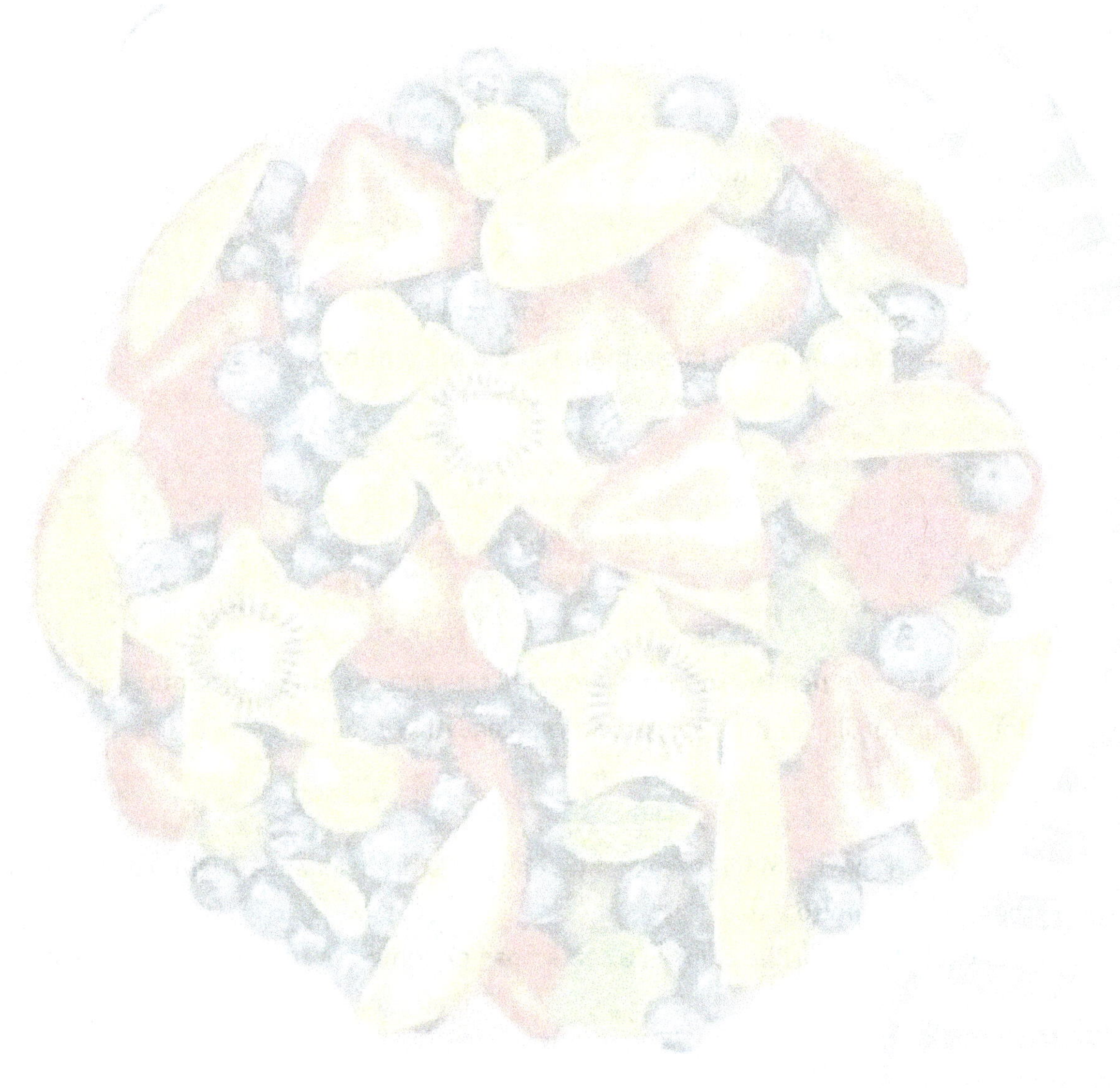

CHAPTER 5

QUICK DESSERTS

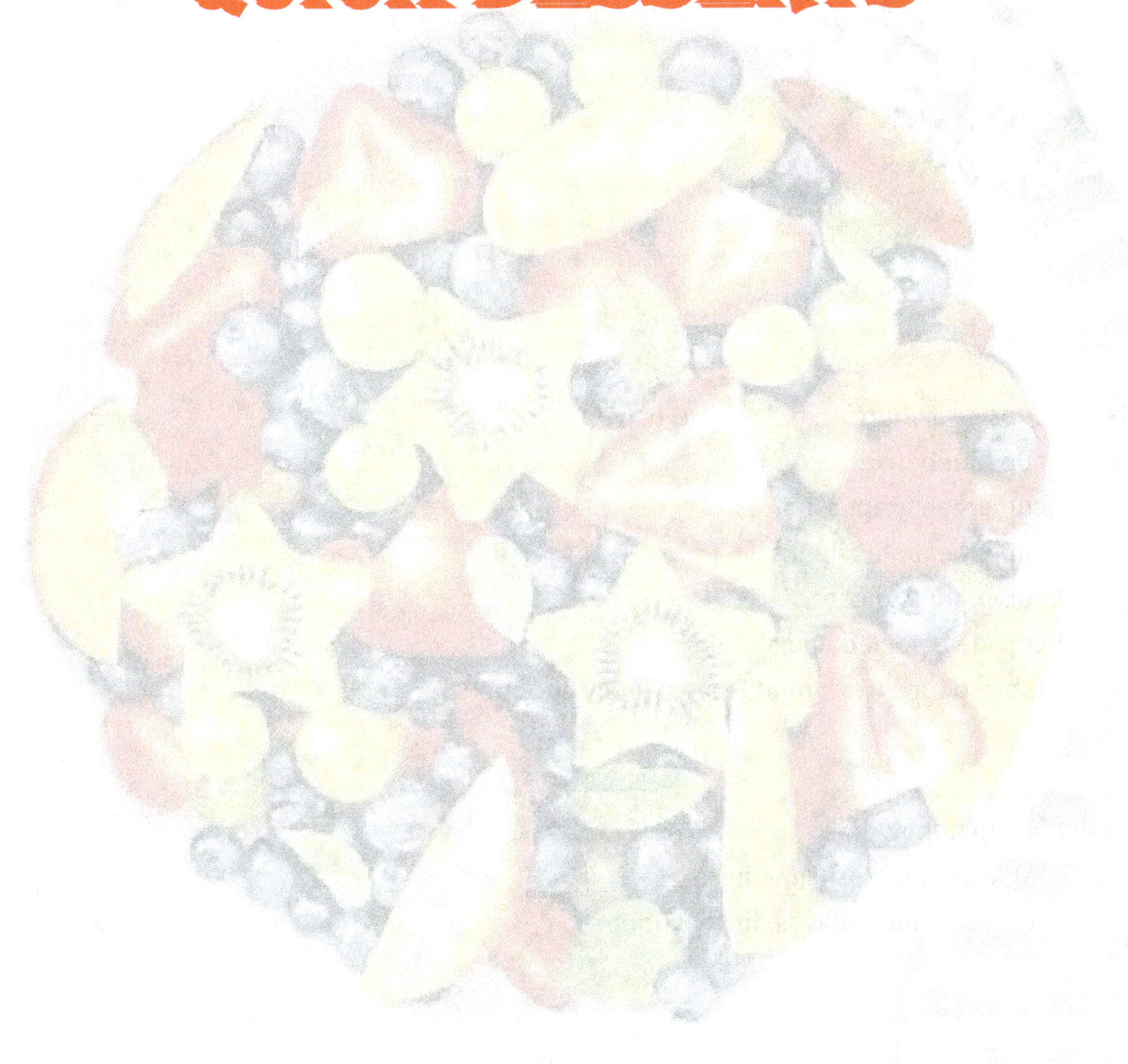

Fruit Salad with Mint

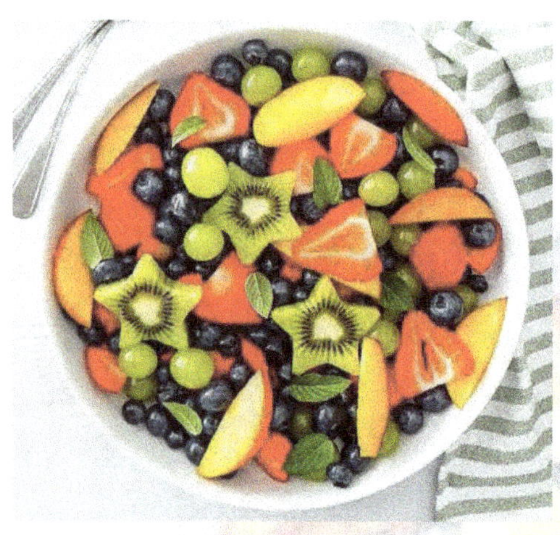

Ingredients:

- 2 cups strawberries, hulled and halved
- 1 cup blueberries
- 1 cup green grapes, halved
- 1 cup pineapple chunks
- 1 cup mango, diced
- 1 cup kiwi, peeled and sliced
- 2 tablespoons fresh mint leaves, finely chopped

Dressing:

- 1/4 cup honey
- 2 tablespoons fresh lime juice
- 1 teaspoon mint leaves, finely chopped

Procedure

- In a large mixing bowl, combine all the fruits and mint leaves.
- In a separate small bowl, whisk together honey, lime juice, and mint for the dressing.
- Pour the dressing over the fruits and gently toss until evenly coated.
- To enable the flavours to mingle, refrigerate for a minimum of half an hour before serving..

- Approximately 15-20 minutes (excluding refrigeration time).

Tips and Tricks:

- Use fresh and ripe fruits for the best flavor.
- Adjust the honey and lime juice quantities according to your sweetness preference.
- Allow the salad to chill for a refreshing taste.

Nutritional Value (per serving):

- Calories: 150 kcal
- Carbohydrates: 38g
- Fiber: 5g
- Vitamin C: 80mg
- Potassium: 300mg

Health Benefits:

- Rich in antioxidants and vitamins.
- Supports immune system and digestion.
- Low in calories and high in fiber.

Packaging and Storing:

- Keep refrigerated in an airtight container..
- Use within two days for optimal flavour and texture.

Estimated Cost of Preparation:

- $15-$20 depending on fruit availability and season.

Precautions:

- Ensure fruits are thoroughly washed.
- Check for allergies before serving.

Post Caution:

- Refrigerate leftovers promptly to avoid spoilage.
- Consume within 2 days for the best taste and texture.

Dark Chocolate-Dipped Strawberries

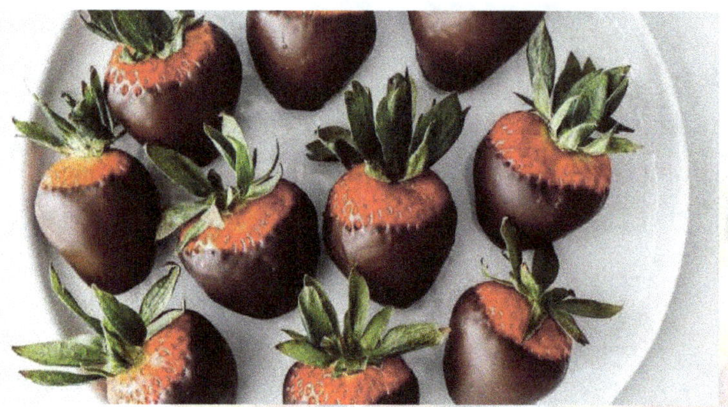

Ingredients:

- 1 pound fresh strawberries, washed and dried
- 8 ounces dark chocolate, finely chopped
- 1 tablespoon coconut oil
- Optional garnishes include shredded coconut, chopped almonds, or sea salt.

Procedure:

- Line a baking sheet with parchment paper.
- In a heatproof bowl, melt the dark chocolate and coconut oil over a double boiler or in short intervals in the microwave, stirring until smooth.
- Holding each strawberry by the stem, dip it into the melted chocolate, allowing excess to drip off.
- Place dipped strawberries on the prepared baking sheet.
- While the chocolate is still wet, immediately sprinkle on the optional toppings.
- Before serving, let the chocolate set at room temperature or in the fridge.

Time of Preparation:

- Approximately 30 minutes (excluding setting time).

Tips and Tricks:

- Ensure strawberries are completely dry to prevent chocolate from seizing.
- Use high-quality dark chocolate for a rich flavor.
- Experiment with toppings for added texture and taste.

- Calories: 120 kcal
- Fat: 8g
- Carbohydrates: 14g
- Fiber: 4g
- Protein: 2g

Health Benefits:

- Antioxidants found in dark chocolate may help heart health.
- Strawberries are rich in vitamin C and contribute to skin health.

Packaging and Storing:

- Place the chocolate-dipped strawberries in a single layer in an airtight container.
- Refrigerate for up to 24 hours for the best taste and texture.

Estimated Cost of Preparation:

- $10-$15 depending on chocolate brand and strawberry availability.

Precautions:

- Avoid getting water into the melted chocolate to prevent seizing.
- Check for nut allergies if using nuts as toppings.

Post Caution:

- Consume within 24 hours for optimal freshness.
- Store in a cool place to prevent chocolate from melting.

Greek Yogurt Popsicles

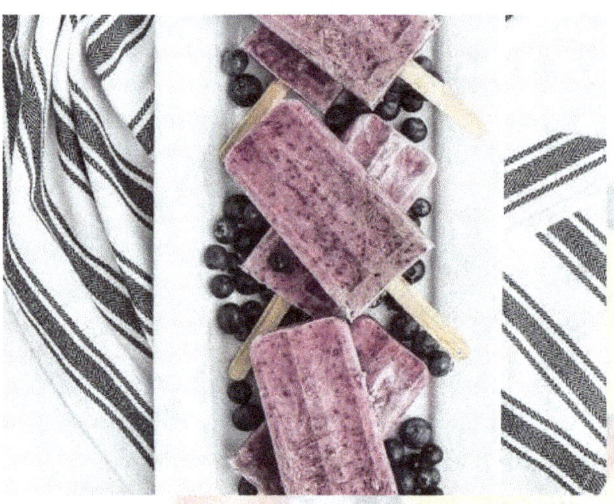

Ingredients:

- 2 cups Greek yogurt
- 1 cup mixed berries (blueberries, raspberries, strawberries)
- 2 tablespoons honey or maple syrup
- 1 teaspoon vanilla extract

Procedure:

- Combine Greek yoghurt, honey (or maple syrup), and vanilla essence in a bowl and stir until thoroughly blended.
- Gently fold in the mixed berries.
- Spoon the mixture into popsicle molds.
- Insert popsicle sticks and freeze for at least 4 hours or until completely solid.
- Run warm water over the moulds for a little while to loosen the popsicles.

Time of Preparation:

- Approximately 10 minutes (excluding freezing time).

Tips and Tricks:

- For a creamier texture, use Greek yoghurt that is full in fat.
- Experiment with different fruit combinations.
- Swirl the mixture in the molds with a toothpick for a marbled effect.

- Calories: 80 kcal
- Protein: 6g
- Carbohydrates: 10g
- Fat: 2g
- Fiber: 1g

Health Benefits:

- Rich in protein, calcium, and probiotics from Greek yogurt.
- Berries provide antioxidants and vitamins.

Packaging and Storing:

- Remove popsicles from molds and store in a freezer-safe bag.
- Consume within 2 weeks for optimal taste.

Estimated Cost of Preparation:

- $5-$8 depending on yogurt brand and berry selection.

Precautions:

- Ensure popsicle sticks are secure in the molds.
- Be cautious when removing popsicles from molds to avoid breakage.

Post Caution:

- Freeze any leftover mixture for a quick batch next time.

CHAPTER 6

ONE-PAN MEALS

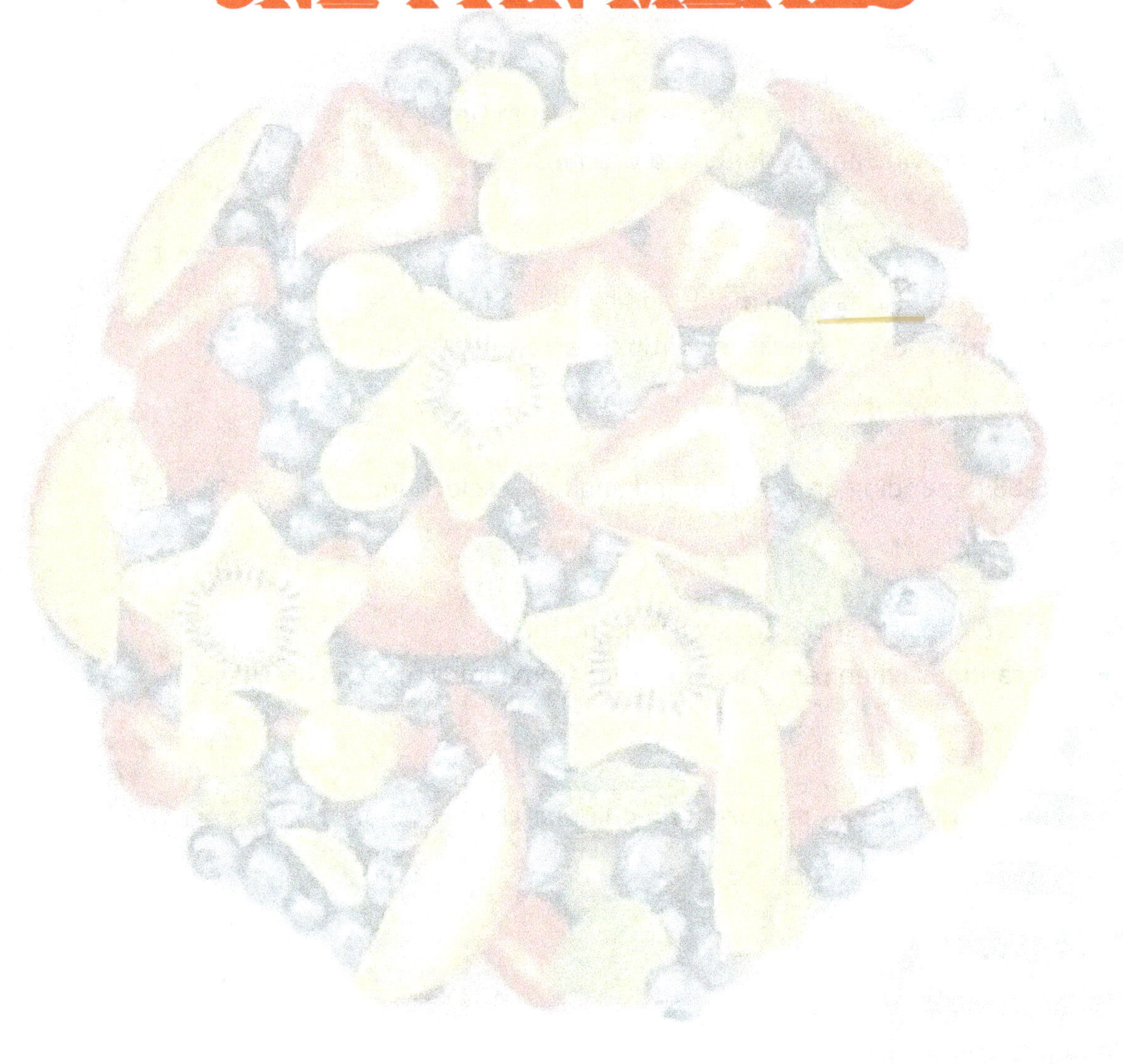

Sheet Pan Lemon Garlic Chicken with Vegetables

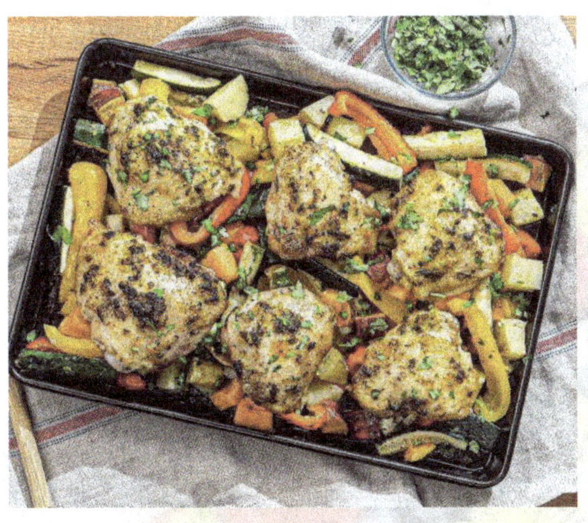

Ingredients:

- 4 boneless, skinless chicken breasts
- 1 pound baby potatoes, halved
- 2 cups baby carrots
- 1 cup broccoli florets
- 1 lemon, thinly sliced
- 4 cloves garlic, minced
- 1/4 cup olive oil
- 2 teaspoons dried oregano
- Salt and pepper to taste
- Fresh parsley for garnish

Procedure:

- Oven Prep: Set the oven's temperature to 400°F, or 200°C.
- Prepare Sheet Pan: Line a large sheet pan with parchment paper or lightly grease it.
- Season Chicken: Place chicken breasts on the sheet pan. Drizzle with olive oil and rub minced garlic, oregano, salt, and pepper over each chicken breast.
- Add Vegetables: Scatter halved baby potatoes, baby carrots, broccoli florets, and lemon slices around the chicken.

- Bake: Bake in the preheated oven for about 25-30 minutes or until the chicken reaches an internal temperature of 165°F (74°C) and vegetables are tender.
- Garnish and Serve: Sprinkle fresh parsley over the dish before serving.

Time of Preparation:

- Approximately 15 minutes for preparation, 25-30 minutes for baking.

Tips and Tricks:

- Ensure even cooking by cutting vegetables to a uniform size.
- For extra flavor, marinate chicken in lemon juice, garlic, and olive oil for 30 minutes before cooking.
- Broil for an additional 2-3 minutes for a golden-brown finish on the chicken.

Nutritional Value (per serving):

- Calories: ~400
- Protein: ~30g
- Carbohydrates: ~25g
- Fat: ~20g

Health Benefits:

- High protein content supports muscle health.
- Rich in vitamins and minerals from vegetables.
- Olive oil provides healthy monounsaturated fats.

Packaging and Storing:

- Remaining food can be kept in the refrigerator for up to three days if it is sealed tightly.
- Reheat in the oven for optimal texture.

Estimated Cost of Preparation:

- $15-$20, depending on ingredient quality and location.

Precautions:

- Ensure chicken reaches a safe internal temperature.
- Be cautious when handling hot pans and utensils.

- Discard leftovers if stored for more than 3 days.
- Consider adjusting portion sizes for dietary needs.

Shrimp and Broccoli Bake

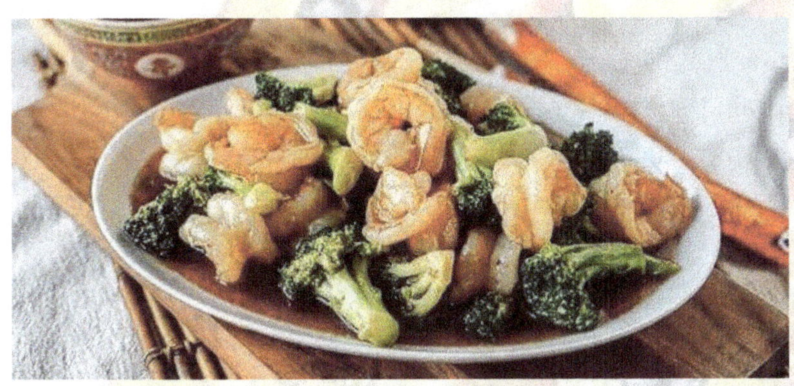

Ingredients:

- 1 pound large shrimp, peeled and deveined
- 4 cups broccoli florets
- 1 cup cherry tomatoes, halved
- 1/2 cup grated Parmesan cheese
- 1/4 cup olive oil
- 4 cloves garlic, minced
- 2 tablespoons lemon juice
- 1 teaspoon dried oregano
- Salt and pepper to taste
- 1/2 cup breadcrumbs (optional for topping)

Procedure:

- Oven Prep: Set the oven's temperature to 375°F, or 190°C.
- Prepare Baking Dish: Grease a baking dish or casserole.

- Prepare Shrimp and Vegetables: In a bowl, combine shrimp, broccoli, cherry tomatoes, minced garlic, olive oil, lemon juice, dried oregano, salt, and pepper. Toss to coat evenly.
- Layer in Baking Dish: Arrange the shrimp and vegetable mixture in the prepared baking dish.
- Top with Cheese (and Breadcrumbs): Sprinkle grated Parmesan cheese over the shrimp and vegetables. Optionally, add a layer of breadcrumbs for a crunchy topping.
- Bake: Bake in the preheated oven for approximately 20-25 minutes or until shrimp are opaque and vegetables are tender.

Time of Preparation:

- Approximately 15 minutes for preparation, 20-25 minutes for baking.

Tips and Tricks:

- Don't overcook shrimp to maintain their tender texture.
- Customize with your favorite herbs or spices for added flavor.
- For a golden crust, broil for the last 2-3 minutes.

Nutritional Value (per serving):

- Calories: ~300
- Protein: ~25g
- Carbohydrates: ~12g
- Fat: ~18g

Health Benefits:

- Lean protein and omega-3 fatty acids are found in prawns.
- Broccoli is rich in fiber, vitamins, and antioxidants.

Packaging and Storing:

- Remaining food can be kept in the refrigerator for up to two days if it is sealed tightly.
- Reheat in the oven or microwave for optimal taste.

Estimated Cost of Preparation:

- $20-$25, depending on the quality of shrimp and other ingredients.

Precautions:

- Ensure shrimp are thoroughly deveined.

- Check for shell remnants in shrimp before cooking.

- Consume leftovers within 2 days to maintain freshness.
- Adjust portion sizes for dietary needs.

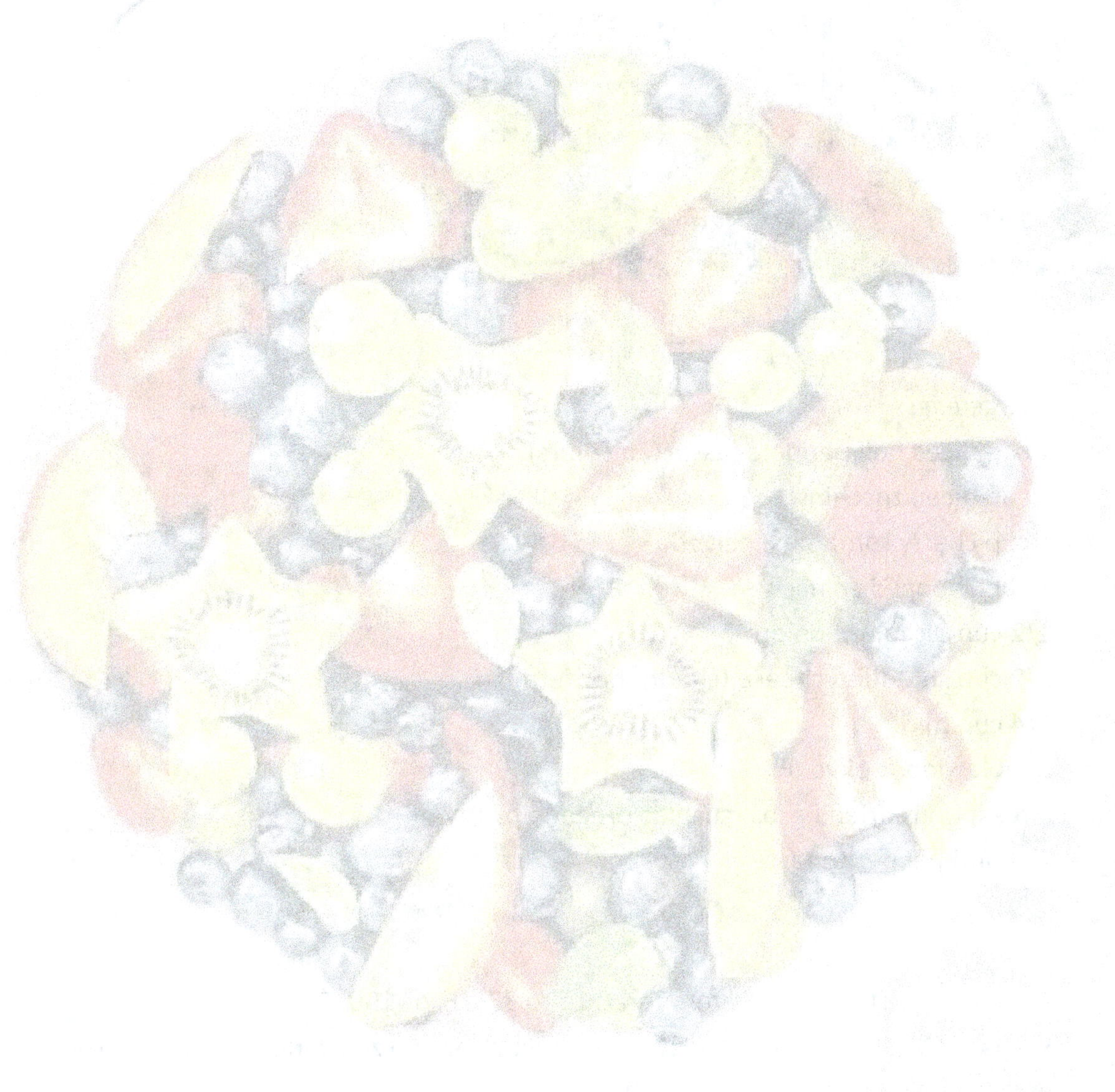

Veggie-Packed Frittata

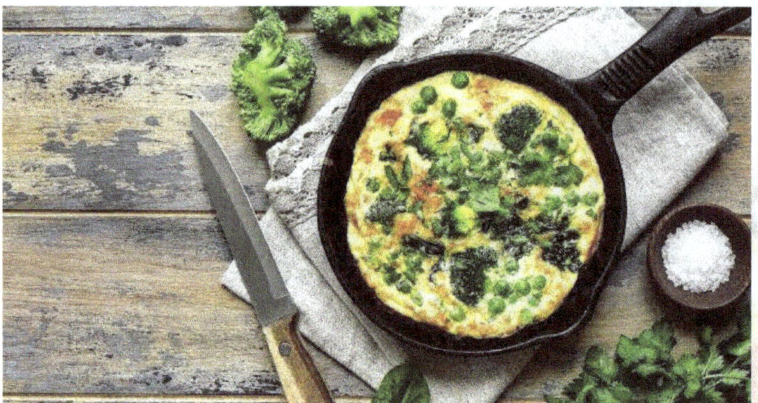

Ingredients:

- 8 large eggs
- 1 cup diced bell peppers (assorted colors)
- 1 cup diced zucchini
- 1 cup cherry tomatoes, halved
- 1 cup chopped spinach
- 1/2 cup diced red onion
- 1/2 cup shredded cheese (cheddar or feta)
- 1/4 cup milk
- 2 tablespoons olive oil
- 2 teaspoons dried herbs (such as oregano or thyme)
- Salt and pepper to taste

Procedure:

- Oven Prep: Set the oven's temperature to 375°F, or 190°C.
- Prepare Vegetables: In a skillet, sauté bell peppers, zucchini, cherry tomatoes, spinach, and red onion in olive oil until softened.
- Whisk Eggs: In a bowl, whisk together eggs, milk, dried herbs, salt, and pepper.
- Combine Ingredients: Add the sautéed vegetables to the whisked eggs. Mix in shredded cheese and combine thoroughly.
- Bake Frittata: Pour the mixture into a greased oven-safe skillet or baking dish. Bake until the centre is set, 20 to 25 minutes.
- Broil (Optional): For a golden top, broil the frittata for an additional 2-3 minutes.

- Approximately 15 minutes for preparation, 20-25 minutes for baking.

Tips and Tricks:

- Use a non-stick skillet for easy removal.
- Experiment with different vegetable combinations.
- Allow the frittata to cool slightly before slicing.

Nutritional Value (per serving):

- Calories: ~180
- Protein: ~12g
- Carbohydrates: ~8g
- Fat: ~12g

Health Benefits:

- High in protein and essential vitamins from eggs.
- Abundance of fiber and antioxidants from veggies.

Packaging and Storing:

- Remaining food can be kept in the refrigerator for up to three days if it is sealed tightly.
- Warm through in the microwave or oven for an easy breakfast or snack.

Estimated Cost of Preparation:

- $10-$15, depending on the cost of vegetables and cheese.

Precautions:

- Ensure eggs are fully cooked to avoid foodborne illness.
- Be cautious when handling hot baking dishes.

Post-Caution:

- Consume within 3 days for optimal freshness.
- Adjust portion sizes to meet dietary requirements.

CHAPTER 8

VEGETARIAN OPTIONS

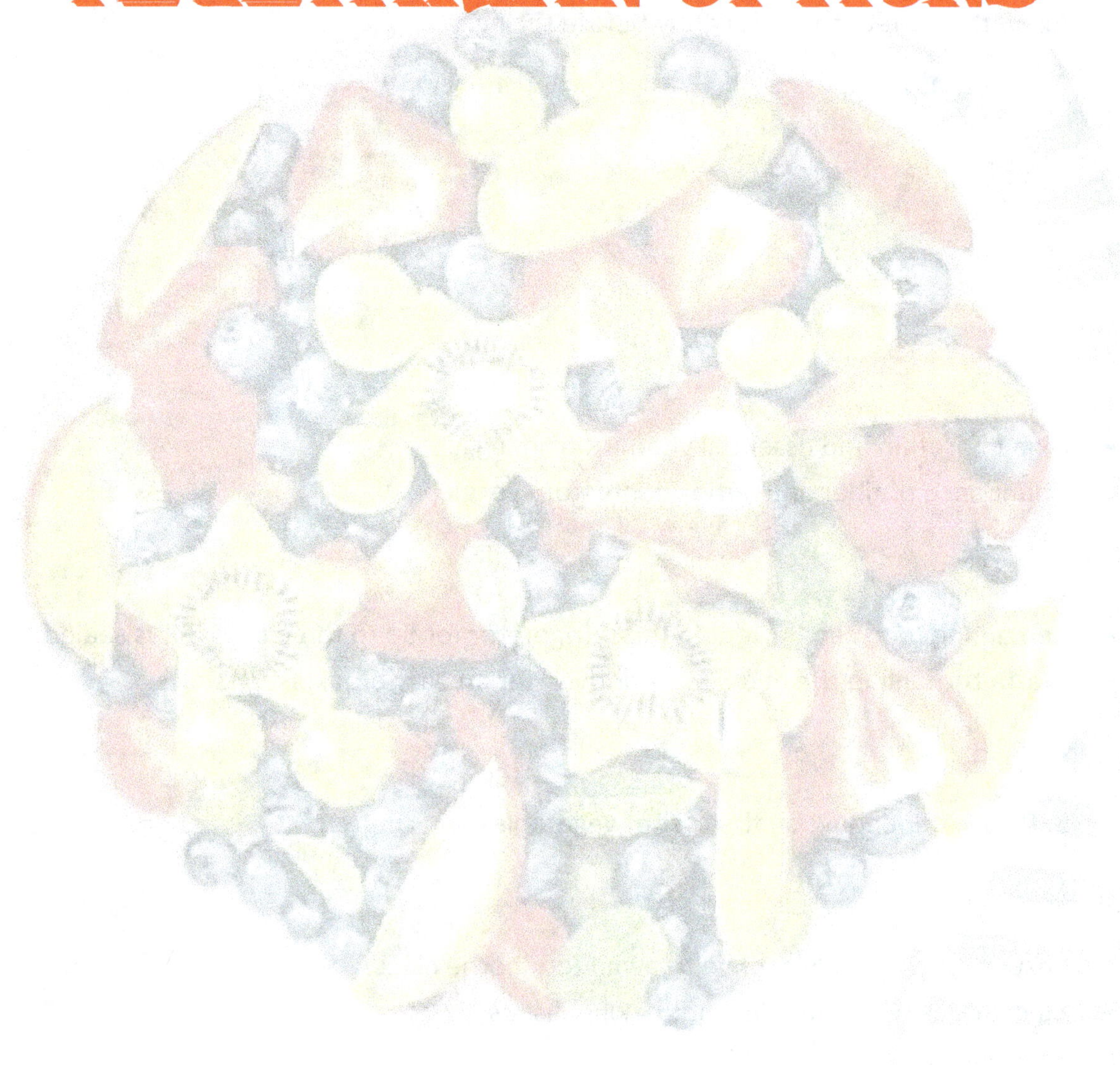

Lentil and Vegetable Stuffed Bell Peppers

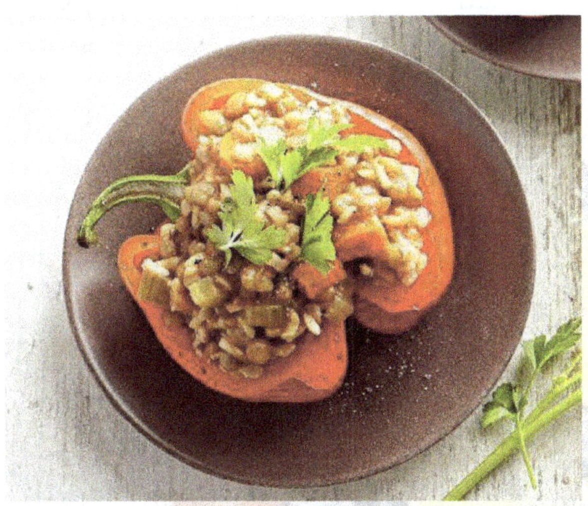

Ingredients:

- 4 large bell peppers (any color)
- 1 cup green lentils, rinsed and drained
- 2 cups vegetable broth
- 1 onion, finely chopped
- 2 cloves garlic, minced
- 1 carrot, grated
- 1 zucchini, diced
- 1 cup cherry tomatoes, halved
- 1 teaspoon dried oregano
- 1 teaspoon cumin
- Salt and pepper to taste
- 2 tablespoons olive oil
- 1 cup shredded mozzarella cheese (optional)

Procedure:

- Preheat the oven to 375°F (190°C).
- Remove the bell peppers' seeds, cut off their tops, and set them aside.
- In a saucepan, combine lentils and vegetable broth. Bring to a boil, then simmer for 20-25 minutes until lentils are tender but not mushy.

- Garlic and onion should be sautéed in olive oil in a skillet until transparent.. Add grated carrot, diced zucchini, and cherry tomatoes. Cook for 5-7 minutes until vegetables are softened.
- Combine sautéed vegetables with cooked lentils. Add oregano, cumin, salt, and pepper. Mix well.
- Stuff each bell pepper with the lentil and vegetable mixture.
- If desired, top each stuffed pepper with shredded mozzarella cheese.
- Place stuffed peppers in a baking dish and bake for 25-30 minutes or until peppers are tender.

Time of Preparation:

- Approximately 1 hour.

Tips and Tricks:

- Choose firm and symmetrical bell peppers for easier stuffing.
- Add the spices and veggies of your choice to the filling..
- To save time, you can pre-cook lentils and prepare filling in advance.

Nutritional Value per Serving (assuming 4 servings):

- Calories: 300
- Protein: 15g
- Fiber: 10g
- Vitamin C: 120% DV
- Iron: 20% DV

Health Benefits:

- Rich in fiber and protein for sustained energy.
- rich in minerals and vitamins from a range of veggies..
- Low in saturated fats, promoting heart health.

Packaging and Storing:

- Remaining food can be kept in the refrigerator for up to three days if it is sealed tightly.
- For a quick meal, reheat in the microwave or oven..

Estimated Cost of Preparation:

- $15-$20

- Ensure lentils are thoroughly cooked to avoid digestive issues.
- Check bell peppers for any signs of spoilage before use.

Post-Caution:

- Monitor individual dietary restrictions or allergies when serving.

Mushroom and Spinach Quiche

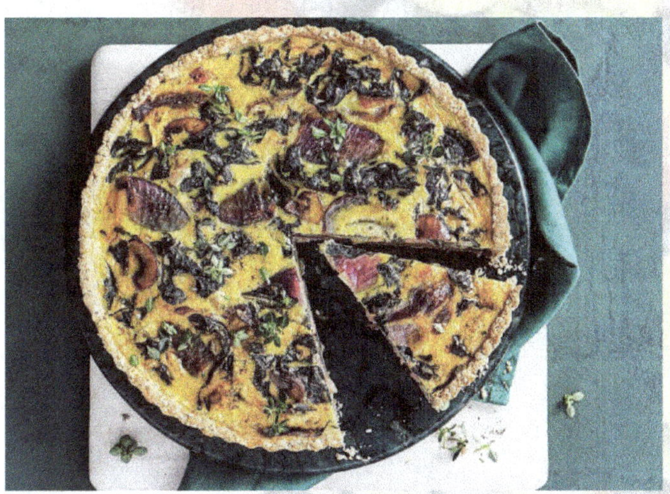

Ingredients:

- 1 pie crust (store-bought or homemade)
- 1 cup sliced mushrooms
- 2 cups fresh spinach, chopped
- 1 small onion, finely chopped
- 3 cloves garlic, minced
- 1 cup shredded Swiss or Gruyere cheese
- 4 large eggs
- 1 cup milk
- Salt and pepper to taste

- 1/2 teaspoon dried thyme
- 1 tablespoon olive oil

Procedure:

- Preheat the oven to 375°F (190°C).
- Place the pie crust in a greased quiche or pie pan.
- Heat the olive oil in a pan over medium heat.. Sauté onions and garlic until softened.
- When the mushrooms begin to release their moisture, add them cut-side down to the skillet.
- Add chopped spinach and cook until wilted. Remove excess moisture if needed.
- In a bowl, whisk together eggs, milk, salt, pepper, and dried thyme.
- Spread the mushroom and spinach mixture over the pie crust. Sprinkle shredded cheese on top.
- Cover the cheese and veggies with the egg mixture.
- Bake for 35 to 40 minutes, or until the top is golden brown and the centre is set, in a preheated oven.

Time of Preparation:

- Approximately 1 hour.

Tips and Tricks:

- Blind bake the pie crust for a few minutes before adding the filling to prevent a soggy crust.
- Experiment with different cheeses like cheddar or feta for varied flavors.
- Allow the quiche to cool for a few minutes before slicing for cleaner cuts.

Nutritional Value per Serving (assuming 6 servings):

- Calories: 280
- Protein: 14g
- Calcium: 20% DV
- Vitamin A: 60% DV
- Iron: 15% DV

Health Benefits:

- Spinach provides essential vitamins and minerals.
- Mushrooms contribute antioxidants and B-vitamins.

- Eggs offer a good source of protein and nutrients.

- Remaining food can be kept in the fridge for up to three days.
- Warm up individual pieces using a microwave or oven..

- $12-$1

- Ensure the eggs are thoroughly cooked to prevent foodborne illness.
- Check the pie crust for any cracks or tears before filling.

- Enjoy this flavorful Mushroom and Spinach Quiche as a versatile meal for breakfast, brunch, or a light dinner.

Spinach and Feta Chickpea Patties

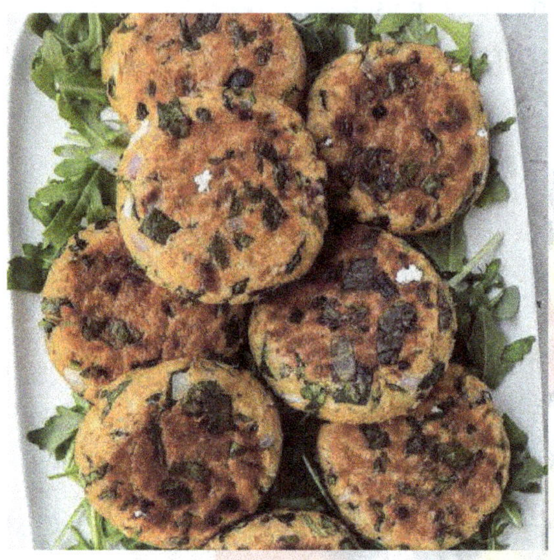

Ingredients:

- Two cans (15 oz each) of rinsed and drained chickpeas
- 2 cups fresh spinach, chopped
- 1/2 cup crumbled feta cheese
- 1/4 cup red onion, finely chopped
- 2 cloves garlic, minced
- 1 teaspoon ground cumin
- 1 teaspoon ground coriander
- 1/2 teaspoon paprika
- Salt and pepper to taste
- 2 tablespoons olive oil
- 1/2 cup breadcrumbs
- 2 large eggs

Procedure:

- In a food processor, combine chickpeas, spinach, feta, red onion, garlic, cumin, coriander, paprika, salt, and pepper. Pulse until a coarse mixture forms.
- Transfer the mixture to a bowl and add breadcrumbs. Mix well.
- Beat the eggs and add them to the chickpea mixture. Stir until combined.
- Form the mixture into patties, approximately 3 inches in diameter.

- In a skillet over medium heat, warm the olive oil. Cook until golden brown, 3–4 minutes per side for the patties.

- Approximately 30 minutes.

- Adjust the spice levels by adding more or less cumin and coriander according to your preference.
- Refrigerate the mixture for 30 minutes before shaping the patties for easier handling.
- For a crispier texture, you can bake the patties in the oven at 375°F (190°C) for 20-25 minutes, flipping halfway.

- Calories: 220
- Protein: 10g
- Fiber: 8g
- Calcium: 15% DV
- Iron: 20% DV

- Chickpeas provide a good source of plant-based protein and fiber.
- Spinach is rich in vitamins A and K.
- Feta adds calcium and a burst of flavor.

- Store any unused mixture or cooked patties in an airtight container in the refrigerator for up to 3 days.
- Reheat in the oven or skillet for a few minutes.

- $10-$12

- Ensure the chickpeas are well-drained to prevent excess moisture in the mixture.
- Watch the cooking time to avoid overcooking and drying out the patties.

- Enjoy these Spinach and Feta Chickpea Patties as a delicious and nutritious alternative to traditional burgers.
- Serve with a side of yogurt sauce or in a whole-grain bun for a complete meal.

CHAPTER 8

LOW-CARB RECIPES

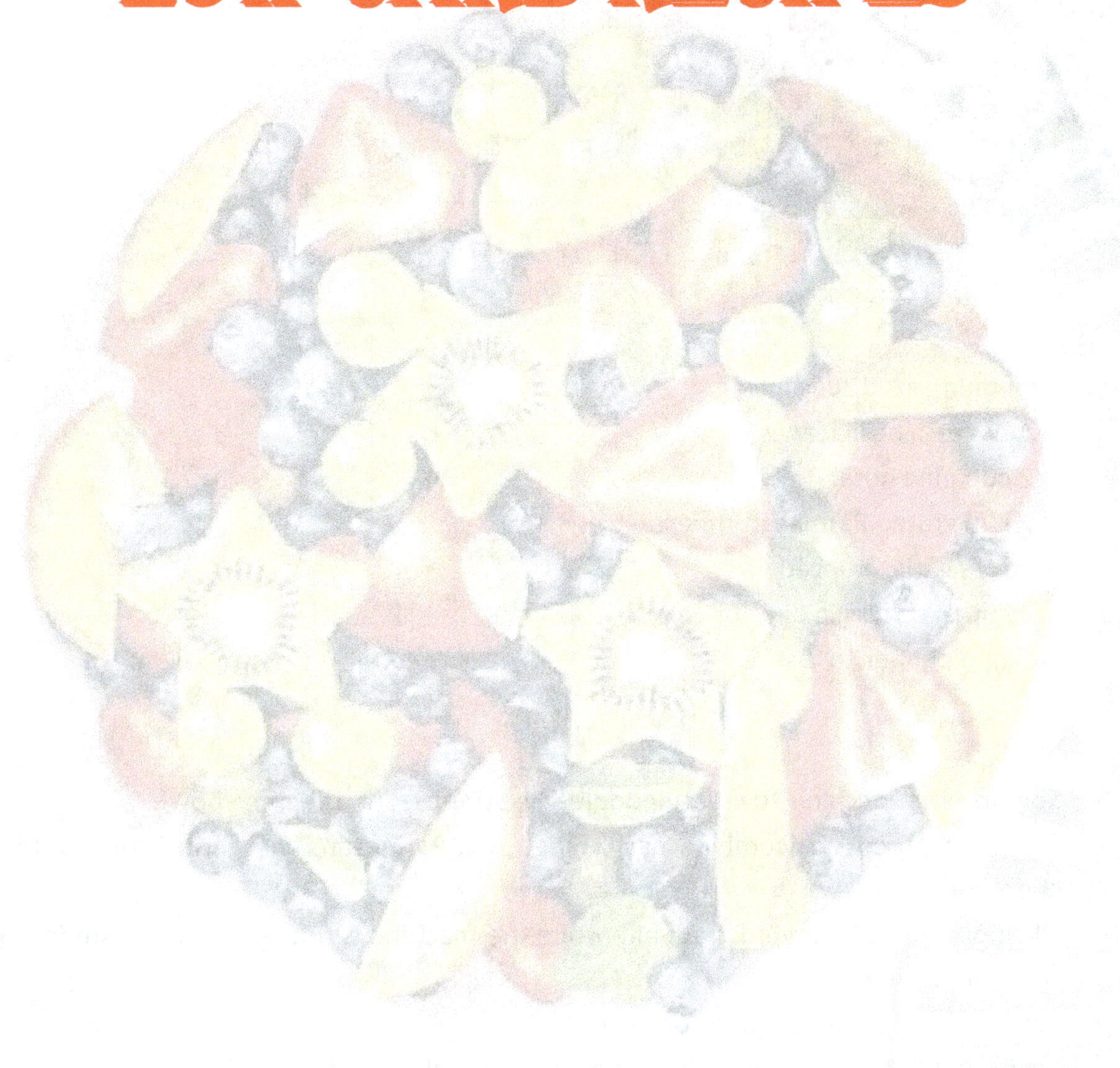

Zucchini Noodles with Pesto

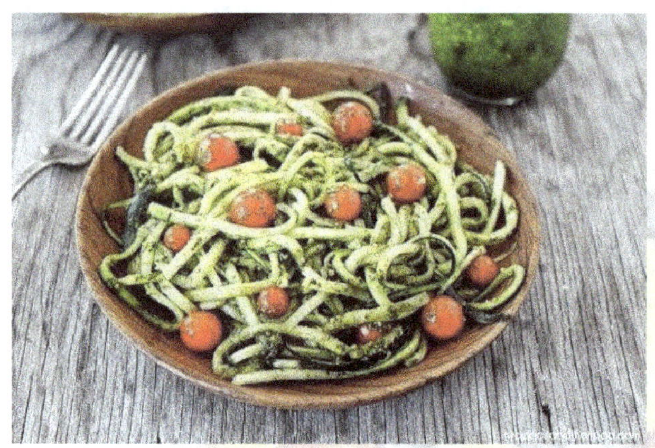

Ingredients:

- 4 medium-sized zucchinis
- 2 cups fresh basil leaves
- 1/2 cup pine nuts
- 1/2 cup grated Parmesan cheese
- 3 cloves garlic, minced
- 1/2 cup extra-virgin olive oil
- Salt and pepper to taste

Procedure:

- Spiralize the zucchinis to create noodle-like strands. Set aside in a bowl.
- In a food processor, combine basil, pine nuts, Parmesan, and garlic. Pulse until finely chopped.
- Olive oil should be added gradually while the machine is operating until a smooth pesto is formed.
- Season with salt and pepper to taste.
- Toss the zucchini noodles with the pesto until well-coated.

Time of Preparation:

- Approximately 15-20 minutes.

- Pat the zucchini noodles dry with a paper towel to remove excess moisture and prevent a watery dish.
- Toast the pine nuts for enhanced flavor.

Nutritional Value (per serving):

- Calories: 250
- Protein: 7g
- Fat: 22g
- Carbohydrates: 9g
- Fiber: 3g

Health Benefits:

- Low in calories and carbohydrates, suitable for a low-carb or keto diet.
- Rich in vitamins A and C from zucchini and basil.
- Healthy fats from olive oil and pine nuts.

Packaging and Storing:

- Store the zucchini noodles and pesto separately.
- Store for up to two days in the refrigerator in sealed containers.

Estimated Cost of Preparation:

- $10-$15 depending on ingredient quality and location.

Precautions:

- Be cautious while using a spiralizer and follow safety guidelines.
- Check for allergies to nuts and adjust the recipe accordingly.

Post-Caution:

- Ensure proper storage to maintain freshness.
- Reheat zucchini noodles briefly to avoid overcooking.

Cauliflower Fried Rice

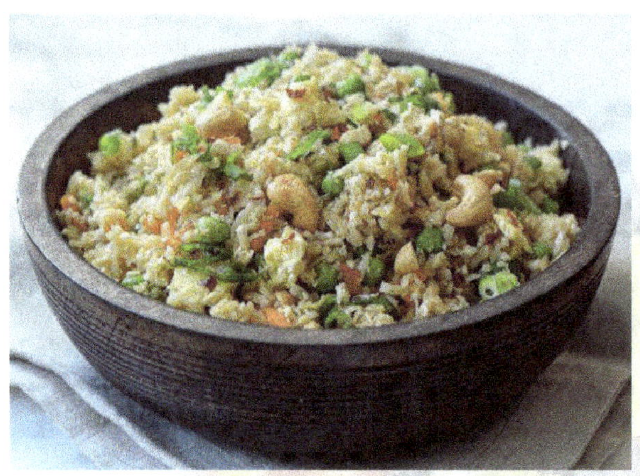

Ingredients

- 1 medium cauliflower, grated
- 2 tablespoons vegetable oil
- 1 cup mixed vegetables (peas, carrots, corn)
- 2 eggs, beaten
- 3 tablespoons soy sauce
- 1 teaspoon sesame oil
- 2 green onions, chopped
- 2 cloves garlic, minced
- 1 teaspoon ginger, grated
- Salt and pepper to taste

Procedure:

- Grate the cauliflower to resemble rice grains. Set aside.
- In a big skillet, heat the vegetable oil over medium heat.
- Add garlic and ginger, sauté until fragrant.
- Add mixed vegetables and cook until softened.
- Place the vegetables on one half of the pan and then transfer the beaten eggs to the other half. . Scramble eggs until cooked.
- Mix in cauliflower rice, soy sauce, and sesame oil. Stir-fry until cauliflower is tender.
- Season with salt and pepper, and garnish with green onions.

- Approximately 20-25 minutes.

Tips and Tricks:

- Ensure the cauliflower is well-drained to avoid a soggy texture.
- Use pre-packaged cauliflower rice for a quicker preparation.

Nutritional Value (per serving):

- Calories: 200
- Protein: 8g
- Fat: 12g
- Carbohydrates: 15g
- Fiber: 6g

Health Benefits:

- Low-carb alternative to traditional fried rice.
- High in fiber and vitamins from cauliflower and vegetables.
- Provides a good source of protein from eggs.

Packaging and Storing:

- For up to three days, store in the refrigerator in sealed containers.
- Warm it up again in a skillet for optimal texture.

Estimated Cost of Preparation:

- $8-$12 depending on ingredient quality and location.

Precautions:

- Be cautious when grating the cauliflower to avoid injuries.
- Ensure the cauliflower is cooked adequately to avoid a raw taste.

Post-Caution:

- Check for freshness before reheating.
- Adjust seasoning if necessary before serving.

Turkey and Vegetable Lettuce Wraps

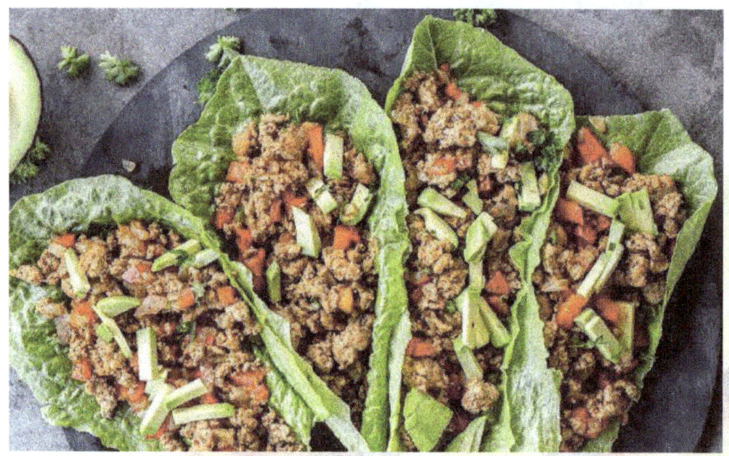

Ingredients:

- 1 lb ground turkey
- 1 tablespoon olive oil
- 1 onion, finely diced
- 2 cloves garlic, minced
- 1 cup bell peppers, diced
- 1 cup carrots, julienned
- 1 cup water chestnuts, chopped
- 1/4 cup soy sauce
- 1 tablespoon hoisin sauce
- 1 teaspoon ginger, grated
- 1 teaspoon sesame oil
- 1 head iceberg or butter lettuce, leaves separated

Procedure:

- Heat the olive oil in a big skillet over medium heat. Cook the ground turkey until it turns brown.
- Add onions and garlic, sauté until softened.
- Stir in bell peppers, carrots, and water chestnuts. Cook until vegetables are tender.
- In a small bowl, mix soy sauce, hoisin sauce, ginger, and sesame oil. Pour over the turkey mixture and stir well.
- Spoon the turkey and vegetable mixture into lettuce leaves, creating wraps.

- Approximately 25-30 minutes.

Tips and Tricks:

- For a healthy option, use ground turkey that is lean.
- Double the vegetable quantity for added nutrition.

Nutritional Value (per serving):

- Calories: 250
- Protein: 20g
- Fat: 12g
- Carbohydrates: 15g
- Fiber: 4g

Health Benefits:

- High in lean protein from turkey.
- rich in minerals and vitamins from vibrant veggies.
- Low-carb and suitable for a keto-friendly diet.

Packaging and Storing:

- Store the turkey and vegetable mixture separately from lettuce leaves.
- Store for up to two days in the refrigerator in sealed containers.

Estimated Cost of Preparation:

- $12-$16 depending on ingredient quality and location.

Precautions:

- Ensure ground turkey is cooked thoroughly.
- Be cautious while chopping vegetables to prevent injuries.

Post-Caution:

- Check the freshness of lettuce leaves before assembling wraps.
- Adjust seasoning if needed before serving.

CHAPTER 9

30-MINUTE MEALS

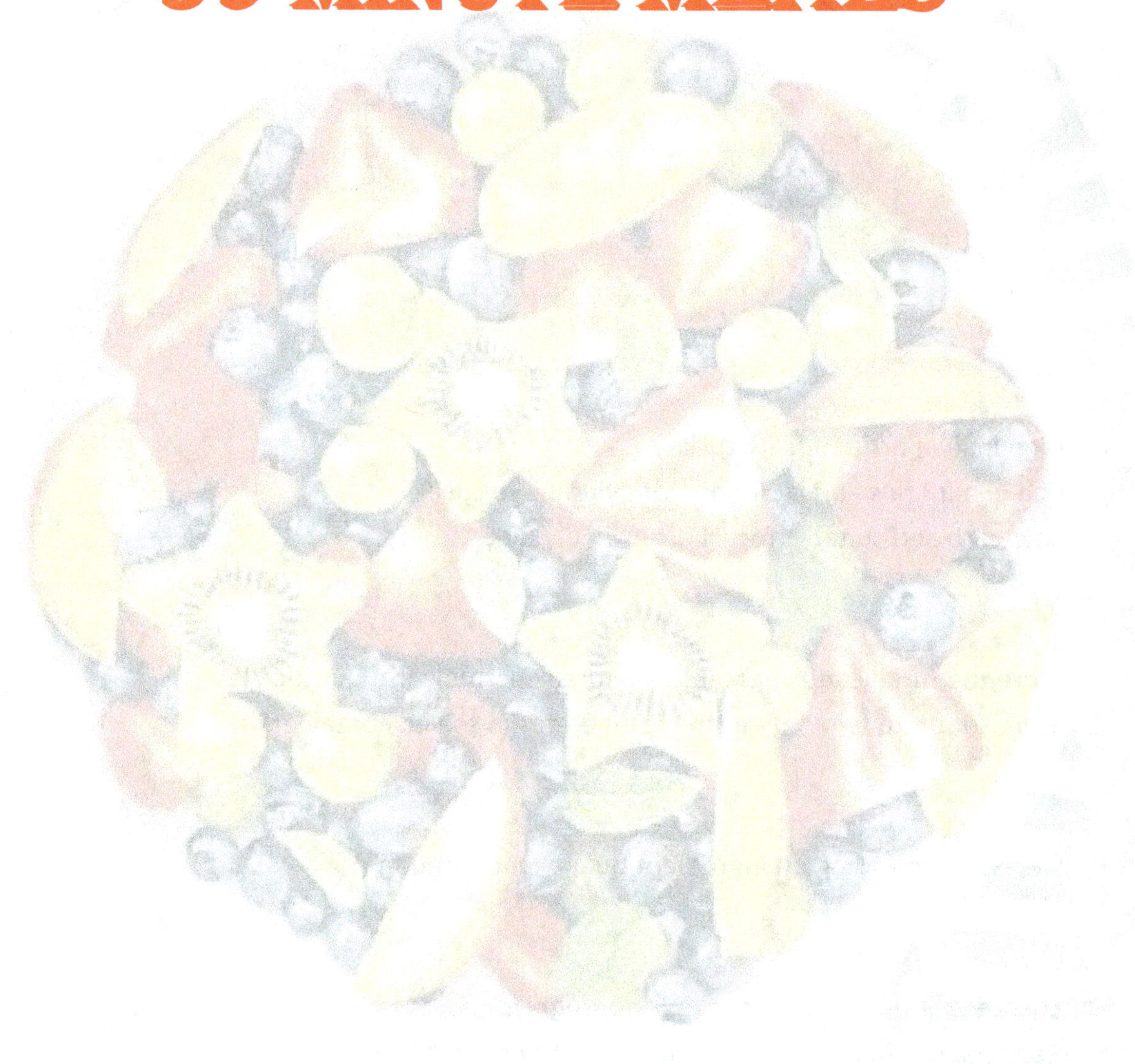

Teriyaki Chicken Bowls

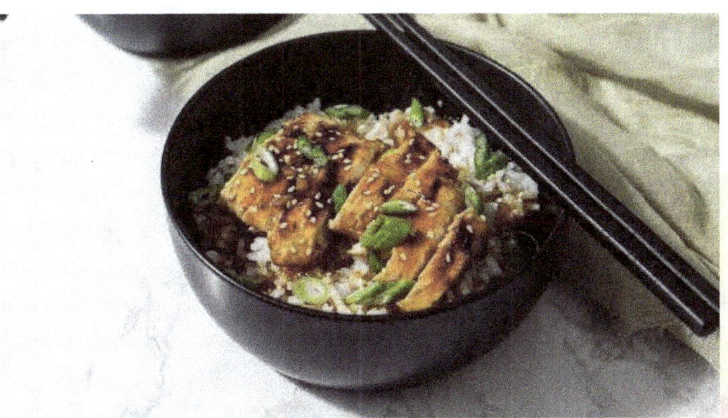

Ingredients:

- One pound of skinless, boneless chicken thighs, cut into small pieces
- 1/2 cup soy sauce
- 1/4 cup mirin (sweet rice wine)
- 2 tablespoons sake (Japanese rice wine)
- 3 tablespoons brown sugar
- 1 tablespoon honey
- 2 cloves garlic, minced
- 1 teaspoon ginger, grated
- 2 tablespoons vegetable oil
- 1 tablespoon cornstarch
- Sesame seeds and green onions for garnish

Procedures:

- In a bowl, mix soy sauce, mirin, sake, brown sugar, honey, garlic, and ginger to create the teriyaki sauce.
- Marinate the chicken pieces in half of the teriyaki sauce for at least 30 minutes.
- In a skillet set over medium-high heat, warm the vegetable oil. When the chicken has marinated, add it and cook it through and browned.
- In a separate pan, bring the remaining teriyaki sauce to a simmer. Thicken sauce by adding cornflour mixture to water.
- Combine the cooked chicken with the thickened teriyaki sauce.
- Serve over rice, garnished with sesame seeds and green onions.

- Approximately 45 minutes, including marinating time.

Tips and Tricks:

- Marinate the chicken for longer for enhanced flavor.
- Adjust sweetness by altering the amount of brown sugar and honey.
- For a smokier flavor, grill the chicken instead of pan-cooking.

Nutritional Value (per serving):

- Calories: ~400
- Protein: ~25g
- Carbohydrates: ~30g
- Fat: ~20g
- Fiber: ~2g

Health Benefits:

- High protein content for muscle health.
- Ginger and garlic may have anti-inflammatory properties.
- Moderation in soy sauce usage for a controlled sodium intake.

Packaging and Storing:

- For up to three days, store in the refrigerator in sealed containers.
- Freeze in portions for longer storage, thawing before reheating.

Estimated Cost of Preparation:

- Approximately $15 for four servings, depending on ingredient quality.

Precautions:

- Ensure chicken is fully cooked to prevent foodborne illnesses.
- Monitor sodium intake due to soy sauce content.

Post Caution:

- Reheat thoroughly to avoid bacterial contamination.
- Discard leftovers after recommended storage times.

Quick and Easy Shrimp Scampi

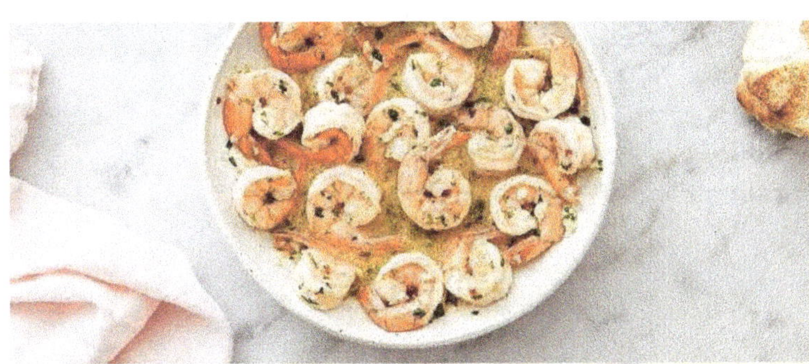

Ingredients:

- 1 pound large shrimp, peeled and deveined
- 8 oz linguine or spaghetti
- 3 tablespoons unsalted butter
- 3 tablespoons olive oil
- 4 cloves garlic, minced
- 1/2 teaspoon red pepper flakes (optional)
- 1/4 cup chicken or vegetable broth
- 1/4 cup dry white wine
- Juice of 1 lemon
- Salt and pepper, to taste
- Fresh parsley, chopped, for garnish
- Grated Parmesan cheese, for serving

Procedures:

- Pasta should be cooked as directed on the package; drain and set aside.
- Melt the butter and olive oil in a big skillet over medium heat.
- Add minced garlic and red pepper flakes (if using), sauté until garlic is fragrant but not browned.
- Add shrimp to the skillet, cook until pink and opaque.
- Pour in chicken or vegetable broth, white wine, and lemon juice. Simmer for 2-3 minutes.
- Season with salt and pepper to taste.
- Toss cooked pasta into the skillet, coating it in the shrimp and sauce mixture.
- Serve with grated Parmesan and garnish with fresh parsley.

- Approximately 20 minutes.

Tips and Tricks:

- Use fresh shrimp for better flavor.
- Adjust spice levels by controlling the amount of red pepper flakes.
- Don't overcook the shrimp to maintain a tender texture.

Nutritional Value (per serving):

- Calories: ~400
- Protein: ~25g
- Carbohydrates: ~30g
- Fat: ~20g
- Fiber: ~2g

Health Benefits:

- Omega-3 fatty acids and minimal calories are found in prawns, making it a protein source.
- Garlic may have antibacterial properties.
- Olive oil contributes to heart health.

Packaging and Storing:

- Remaining food can be kept in the refrigerator for up to two days if it is sealed tightly.
- Reheat gently to avoid overcooking the shrimp.

Estimated Cost of Preparation:

- Approximately $20 for four servings, depending on ingredient quality.

Precautions:

- Ensure shrimp is fully cooked to prevent foodborne illnesses.
- Be cautious with salt, considering the salt content in Parmesan.

Post Caution:

- Consume leftovers promptly.
- Reheat thoroughly to maintain food safety.

Beef and Broccoli Stir-Fry

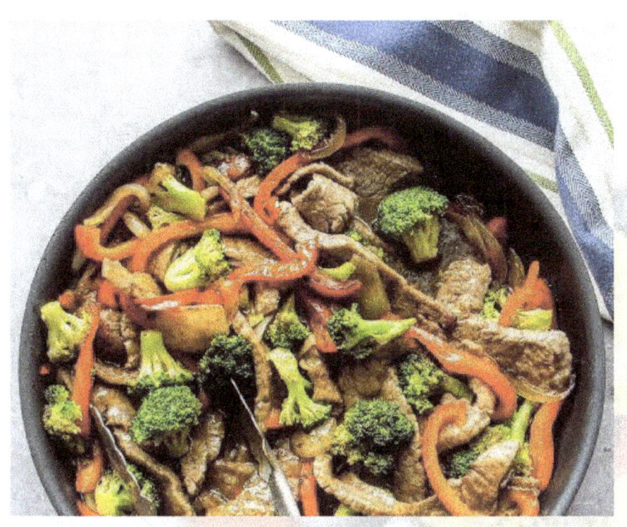

Ingredients:

- 1 pound flank steak, thinly sliced
- 1/2 cup soy sauce
- 3 tablespoons oyster sauce
- 2 tablespoons hoisin sauce
- 1 tablespoon cornstarch
- 2 tablespoons vegetable oil
- 4 cups broccoli florets
- 3 cloves garlic, minced
- 1 tablespoon fresh ginger, grated
- 2 tablespoons sesame oil
- 2 green onions, sliced
- Sesame seeds for garnish (optional)
- Cooked white rice for serving

Procedures:

- In a bowl, mix soy sauce, oyster sauce, hoisin sauce, and cornstarch to create the marinade.
- Marinate sliced beef in half of the marinade for at least 30 minutes.
- In a big skillet or wok, heat the vegetable oil over high heat. Stir-fry marinated beef until browned; set aside.

- In the same pan, stir-fry broccoli, garlic, and ginger until broccoli is crisp-tender.
- Add the cooked beef back to the pan and pour in the remaining marinade. Stir to combine.
- Drizzle sesame oil over the stir-fry and toss to coat.
- Add sesame seeds and sliced green onions as garnish.
- Serve over cooked white rice.

Time of Preparation:

- Approximately 30 minutes, including marinating time.

Tips and Tricks:

- Slice beef against the grain for tenderness.
- Blanch broccoli before stir-frying for a vibrant color.
- Customize the sauce's sweetness and saltiness to taste.

Nutritional Value (per serving):

- Calories: ~400
- Protein: ~30g
- Carbohydrates: ~20g
- Fat: ~20g
- Fiber: ~5g

Health Benefits:

- High protein content supports muscle health.
- Broccoli provides vitamins, minerals, and fiber.
- Ginger and garlic may have anti-inflammatory properties.

Packaging and Storing:

- For up to three days, store in the refrigerator in sealed containers.
- Reheat gently to maintain the beef's texture.

Estimated Cost of Preparation:

- Approximately $25 for four servings, depending on ingredient quality.

Precautions:

- Ensure beef is fully cooked to prevent foodborne illnesses.
- Be cautious with sodium intake due to soy and oyster sauce.

- Consume leftovers promptly.
- Reheat thoroughly to maintain food safety.
- Enjoy your flavorful Beef and Broccoli Stir-Fry!

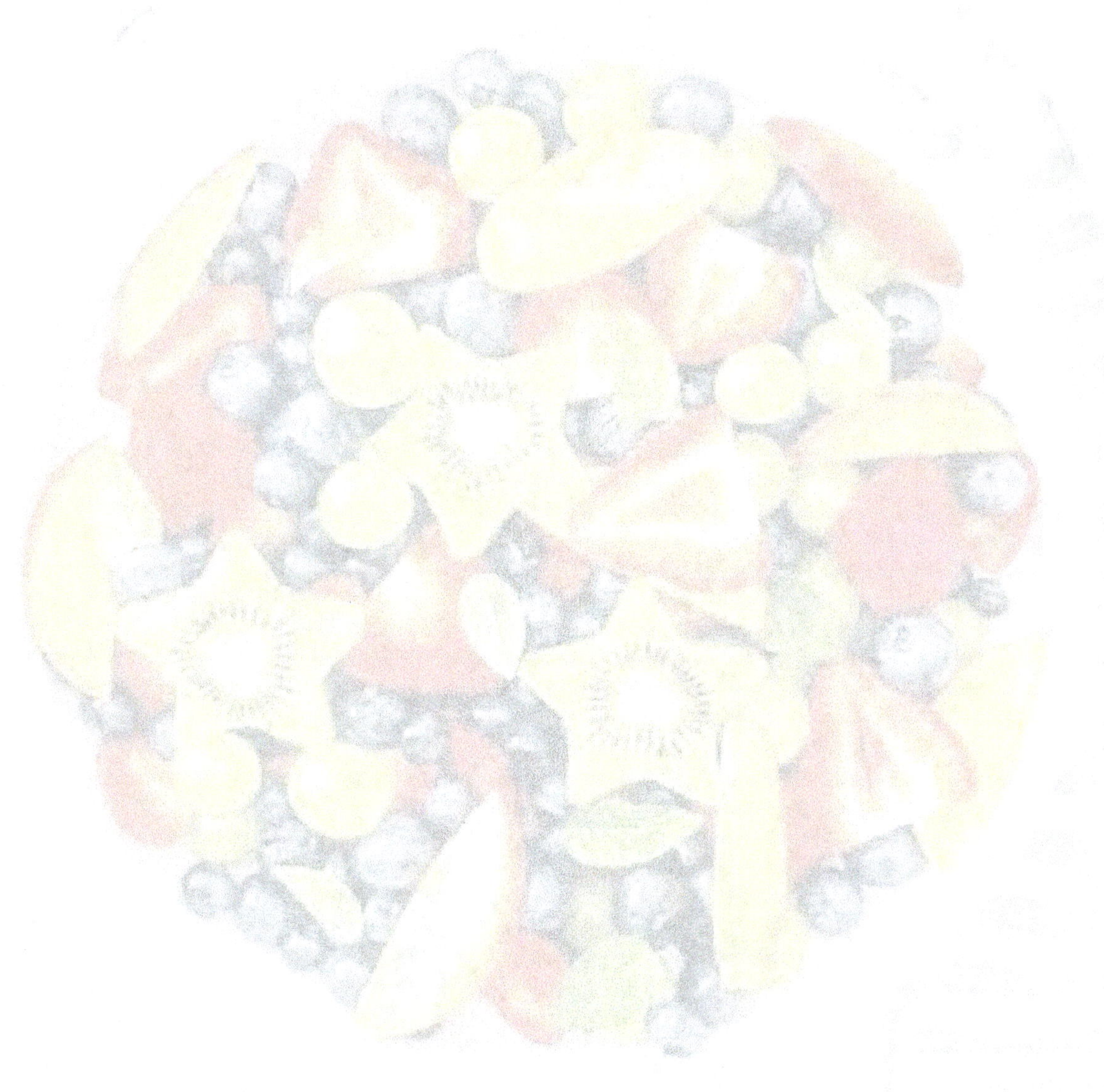

CHAPTER 10

MAKE-AHEAD FREEZER MEALS

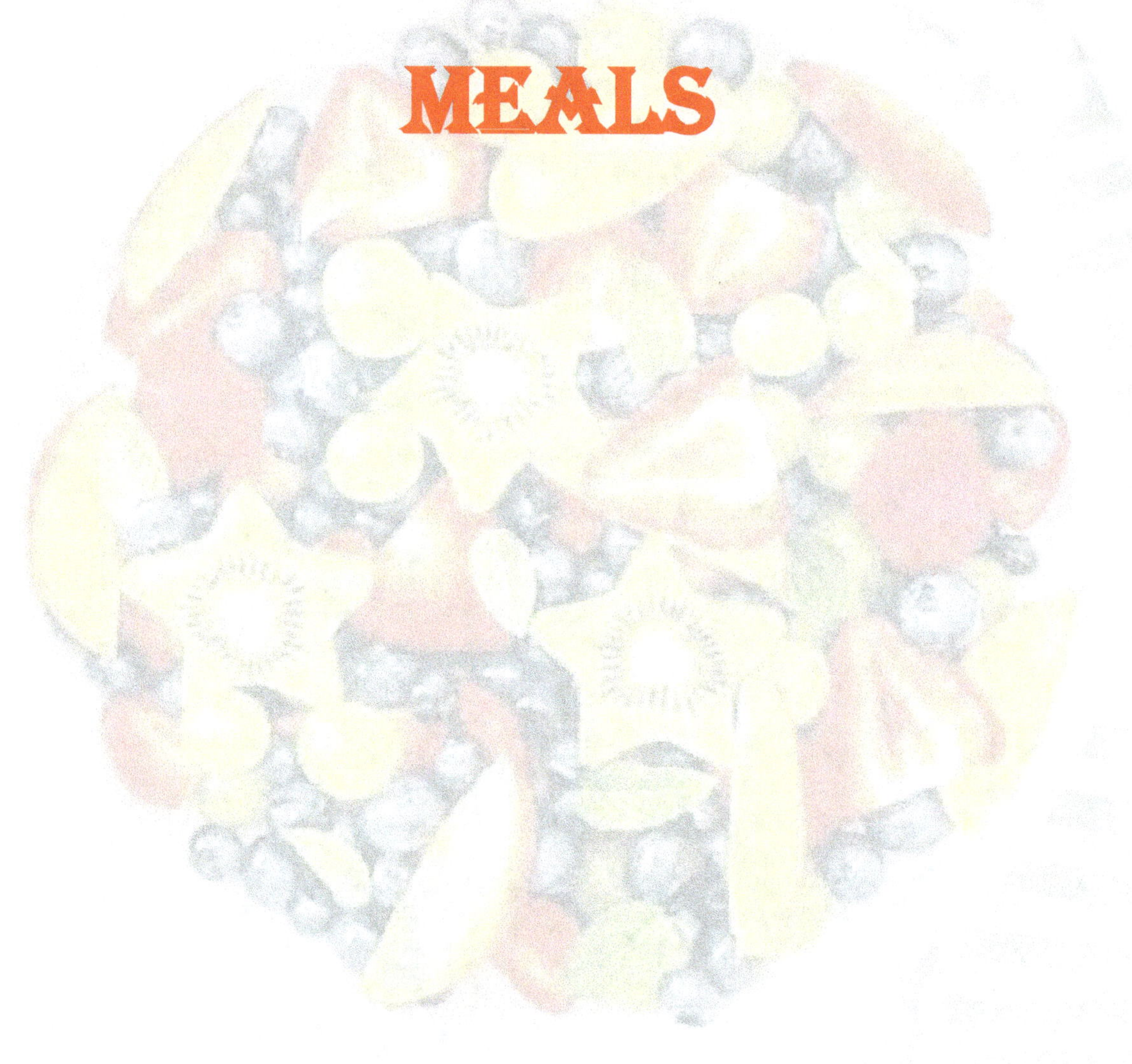

Chicken and Rice Casserole

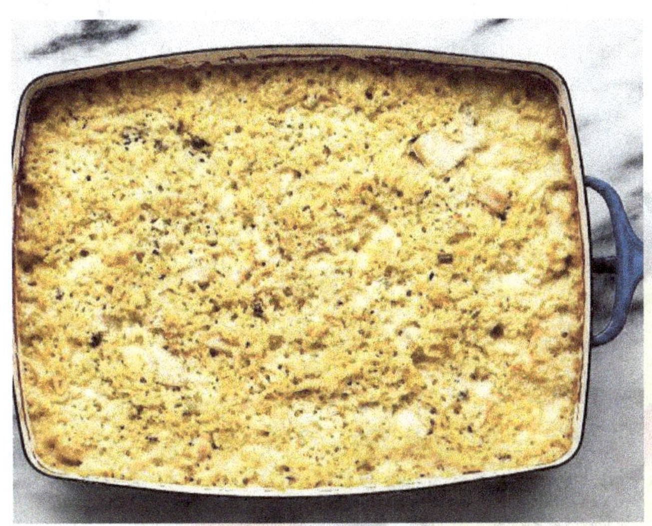

Ingredients:

- 2 cups cooked chicken, shredded
- 1 cup white rice, uncooked
- 1 onion, diced
- 1 bell pepper, chopped
- 1 cup frozen peas
- 2 cloves garlic, minced
- 1 can (10.5 oz) cream of mushroom soup
- 1 cup chicken broth
- 1 cup shredded cheddar cheese
- 1 teaspoon dried thyme
- Salt and pepper to taste
- 2 tablespoons olive oil

Procedure:

- Preheat the oven to 375°F (190°C).
- Heat the olive oil in a big skillet over medium heat. . Sauté onions, bell pepper, and garlic until softened.
- Add uncooked rice to the skillet and stir to coat with oil.
- In a separate bowl, mix cream of mushroom soup and chicken broth until well combined.

- In a greased baking dish, combine cooked chicken, rice mixture, frozen peas, soup mixture, thyme, salt, and pepper. Mix thoroughly.
- Top with shredded cheddar cheese.
- Bake the baking dish for thirty minutes with the foil covering it. After removing the foil, bake the cheese for a further fifteen minutes, or until it is bubbling and melted.
- Before serving, let it a few minutes to rest.

Time of Preparation:

- Approximately 1 hour.

Tips and Tricks:

- Use rotisserie chicken for added flavor and convenience.
- For a fiery kick, add a small amount of hot sauce or cayenne pepper.
- Customize with your favorite vegetables like carrots or broccoli.

Nutritional Value (Per Serving):

- Calories: ~400
- Protein: ~25g
- Carbohydrates: ~35g
- Fat: ~18g

Health Benefits:

- High in protein, which promotes the growth and repair of muscles.
- Provides essential vitamins and minerals from vegetables.
- Balanced carbohydrates for sustained energy.

Packaging and Storing:

- Allow the casserole to cool completely before storing.
- Divide into airtight containers and refrigerate for up to 3 days.
- Freeze for longer storage, up to 2-3 months.

Estimated Cost of Preparation:

- $15-$20 (varies based on ingredient quality and location).

Precautions:

- Ensure chicken is thoroughly cooked to an internal temperature of 165°F (74°C).

- Check for food allergies among consumers.

Post-Caution:

- Reheat leftovers to at least 165°F (74°C).
- Any leftovers that have been left out for longer than two hours should be thrown out.

Vegetarian Lasagna Roll-Ups

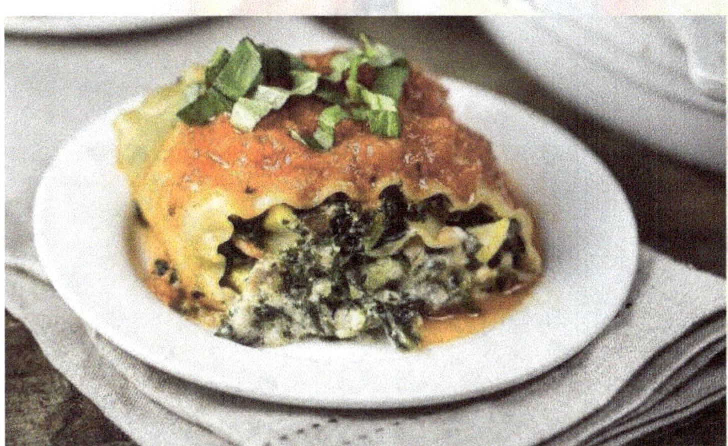

Ingredients:

- 12 lasagna noodles
- 2 cups ricotta cheese
- 1 cup shredded mozzarella cheese
- 1 cup grated Parmesan cheese
- 1 egg, beaten
- 1 cup fresh spinach, chopped
- 1 cup marinara sauce
- 1 teaspoon dried oregano
- 1 teaspoon garlic powder
- Salt and pepper to taste
- Fresh basil for garnish

- Cook lasagna noodles according to package instructions. Drain and set aside.
- In a bowl, combine ricotta, mozzarella, Parmesan, beaten egg, chopped spinach, oregano, garlic powder, salt, and pepper.
- Lay out cooked lasagna noodles and spread the cheese mixture evenly over each noodle.
- Roll up the noodles and place them seam-side down in a baking dish.
- Pour marinara sauce over the roll-ups and sprinkle with additional mozzarella and Parmesan cheese.
- Bake at 375°F (190°C) for 20-25 minutes, or until the cheese is melted and bubbly.
- Garnish with fresh basil before serving.

Time of Preparation:

- Approximately 45 minutes.

Tips and Tricks:

- Use no-boil lasagna noodles for quicker preparation.
- Try a variety of cheese combinations to add more taste.
- Add sautéed mushrooms or diced bell peppers for extra veggies.

Nutritional Value (Per Serving):

- Calories: ~350
- Protein: ~15g
- Carbohydrates: ~30g
- Fat: ~18g

Health Benefits:

- High protein content from ricotta and mozzarella.
- Spinach provides iron, vitamins, and antioxidants.
- Lower saturated fat compared to traditional meat lasagna.

Packaging and Storing:

- Allow the roll-ups to cool before storing.
- For up to three days, keep in the refrigerator in an airtight container.
- Reheat in the oven or microwave.

- $10-$15 (may vary based on ingredient quality and location).

Precautions:

- Ensure the spinach is thoroughly washed.
- Check for egg allergies among consumers.

Post-Caution:

- Reheat leftovers to at least 165°F (74°C).
- Any leftovers that have been left out for longer than two hours should be thrown out.

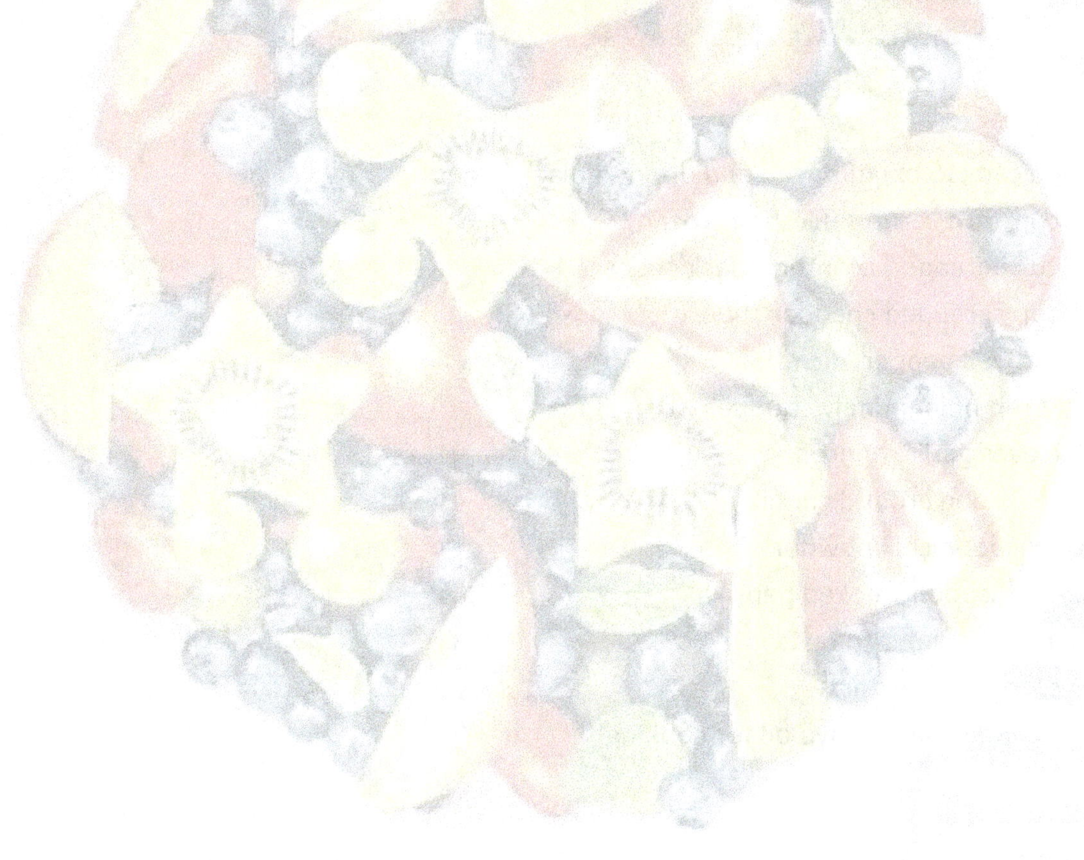

Black Bean and Corn Quesadillas

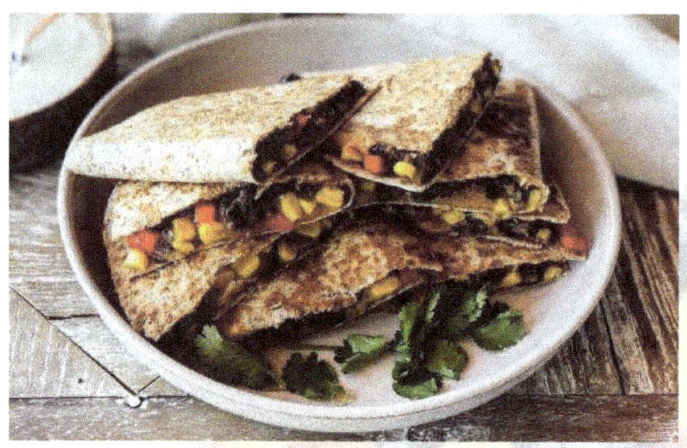

Ingredients:

- One can (15 oz) of rinsed and drained black beans
- 1 cup corn kernels (fresh or frozen)
- 1 cup shredded Monterey Jack cheese
- 1 cup shredded cheddar cheese
- 1 red bell pepper, diced
- 1/2 red onion, finely chopped
- 2 cloves garlic, minced
- 1 teaspoon ground cumin
- 1 teaspoon chili powder
- 1/2 teaspoon smoked paprika
- Salt and pepper to taste
- 8 small flour tortillas
- Cooking spray or olive oil for cooking

Procedure:

- In a bowl, mix black beans, corn, cheeses, diced bell pepper, red onion, minced garlic, cumin, chili powder, smoked paprika, salt, and pepper.
- Lay out the tortillas and spread the black bean and corn mixture evenly over half of each tortilla.
- Fold the tortillas in half, creating quesadillas.
- Heat a skillet over medium heat and lightly coat with cooking spray or olive oil.

- Cook until the cheese is melted and the quesadillas are golden brown, 2 to 3 minutes per side.
- Repeat until all quesadillas are cooked.
- Cut into wedges and serve with your favorite salsa or guacamole.

Time of Preparation:

- Approximately 20 minutes.

Tips and Tricks:

- Customize with additional veggies like diced tomatoes or jalapeños.
- Add cooked chicken or tofu for extra protein.
- Use a non-stick skillet for easier flipping.

Nutritional Value (Per Serving):

- Calories: ~300
- Protein: ~12g
- Carbohydrates: ~40g
- Fat: ~10g

Health Benefits:

- Rich in fiber from black beans and corn.
- Provides a good source of vitamins and minerals from vegetables.
- Balanced combination of protein and carbohydrates.

Packaging and Storing:

- Allow quesadillas to cool before storing.
- Wrap individually in foil or plastic wrap.
- For extended storage, freeze or refrigerate for up to two days.

Estimated Cost of Preparation:

- $8-$12 (may vary based on ingredient quality and location).

Precautions:

- Ensure beans are thoroughly rinsed to reduce sodium content.
- Check for any allergies to peppers or spices among consumers.

- Reheat leftovers to at least 165°F (74°C).
- Any leftovers that have been left out for longer than two hours should be thrown out.

CONCLUSION

In conclusion, the "Easy Quick Healthy Meal Prep Cookbook" serves as a valuable resource for individuals seeking convenient and nutritious meal options. The cookbook not only provides a diverse range of recipes but also emphasizes efficiency, making it suitable for busy lifestyles. Its focus on healthy ingredients and straightforward preparation methods encourages a balanced approach to nutrition without compromising on taste. By promoting easy meal prepping strategies, this cookbook empowers readers to maintain a sustainable and health-conscious approach to their dietary habits. Overall, it is a practical guide that aligns with the growing need for accessible and time-efficient solutions in the realm of healthy cooking.

www.ingramcontent.com/pod-product-compliance
Lightning Source LLC
Chambersburg PA
CBHW080725260726
48660CB00010B/3695